Fully Fertile

A 12-week plan for optimal fertility

TAMARA QUINN, ELISABETH HELLER & JEANIE LEE BUSSELL

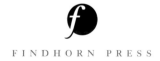

FINDHORN PRESS

The rights of Tamara Quinn, Elisabeth Heller, and Jeanie Lee Bussell to be identified as the authors of this work have been asserted by them in accordance with the Copyright, Designs and Patents Act 1998.

First published by Findhorn Press 2008

ISBN: 978-1-84409-124-9

British Library Cataloguing-in-Publication Data. A catalogue record for this book is available from the British Library.

Cover designed by Damian Keenan
Book designed by The Bridgewater Book Company
Printed and bound by C&C Offset, China

1 2 3 4 5 6 7 8 9 10 11 12 13 14 13 12 11 10 09 08

Published by
Findhorn Press
305A The Park,
Findhorn, Forres IV36 3TE
Scotland, United Kingdom

Tel +44-(0)1309-690582
Fax +44(0)1309-690036
eMail: info@findhornpress.com
www.findhornpress.com

Jeanie, Beth and Tami would like to acknowledge the following individuals for their support, faith, and assistance in the creation of this book:

Jason Bussell, Matt Heller, Brian Quinn, Kevin and Courtney Quinn, Georgia, Jackson and Calvin Heller, Lorraine and Joseph Bilich, Tom and Jackie Timko, Goswami Kriyananda and the Temple of Kriya Yoga, Liz and John Heller, Hahlmohni, Um-ma and Ah-pah, Carol Thorne, Barb and Bill Quinn, Bussell and Lee Families, Dr. Huiyan Cai, Yogarupa Rod Stryker, The Physicians at Fertility Centers of Illinois, Penny Baxter, Lori Butler, Marie Davidson, Howard Hamilton, Trish Nealon, Mary Rowles, Dottie Jeffries, Thierry Bogliolo, Dr. Laura Berman, Stuart-Rodgers Photography, and Paulette Hicks.

We would also like to extend a heartfelt thanks to all of our students and patients at Pulling Down the Moon who inspire us everyday.

Note:

Before applying any techniques described in this or any other nutrition, exercise, or holistic program, an individual should always consult and obtain professional medical advice, including from their doctor.

Not all of the techniques and exercises in this book may be suitable for all readers, and this and any other exercise program may result in physical injury. Women, whether pregnant or not, or men undergoing treatment for infertility should consult their doctor before beginning any exercise, yoga, or holistic program.

The patient-specific details, stories and narratives in this book have been altered to protect the patients' confidentiality. Names and identifying characteristics of the people have been changed. Specific references to websites, books, or videos do not constitute an endorsement by the authors or the publisher.

Section One: **The Physical Practices**

Section Two: **A Fertile Mind**

Section Three: **The Esoteric Tools (Spirit)**

Introduction

Beth and Tami write:

They say that when the universe has a need, it manifests in many minds at the same time... or at least two. That was the case in the "birth" of Pulling Down the Moon. Tami and Beth were at a yoga center on Chicago's north shore when Tami asked if Beth could teach private yoga to a friend of hers—a woman who was having trouble getting pregnant. Unfortunately, the woman was also her children's teacher so working with her on such a sensitive issue felt a little too close for comfort. Beth was recovering from the stillbirth of her daughter, Georgia, and gathering her courage to re-enter the trying-to-conceive trenches. Beth had trouble getting pregnant with Georgia, and had used yoga extensively during the process. What Tami didn't know was that she had recently written a thesis on yoga for fertility and was planning to offer a fertility yoga class at the local studio where they both taught yoga. When she mentioned this to Tami, Tami's jaw dropped.

"But I was going to offer a fertility yoga class," she said. "I've been working on it for months!"

For a moment they just looked at each other, each sizing the other up. Then the teacher called everyone to their mats. Class was starting.

"Well," they said, "let's talk about it after class."

After class they started to share their thoughts on how yoga could help support fertility. Although Beth knew Tami had twins, she didn't realize that Tami was a former fertility patient, too. Their views were so remarkably similar that in the end they decided to join forces and work on a class together. They met for tea later in the week and began to dream about what they wanted to create...

*It would be more than a yoga class. They wanted a place where women could come and learn about yoga philosophy and experience traditional healing methods with practitioners who specialized in fertility. They would have a tea room that would be the antithesis of a doctor's waiting room. There'd be incense and candles burning, soft music, and beautiful things to look at. **More than anything else... everyone there would get it.** They'd get the shots, the anxiety, the ovulation predictor kits; they'd get the misery of receiving another* *baby shower invitation or another unsuccessful cycle... And it would be called... it would be called...*

What would it be called?

After several cups of tea they recalled a meditation entitled "Pulling Down the Moon." It focused on discovering the divine nature of our true selves.

"That's it," they said simultaneously. "That's the name of the class."

The words "pulling down the moon" resonated with so many symbols from Eastern and Western spiritual beliefs that they felt it spoke volumes in one simple phrase. The moon, as we all know, is intimately related to the tides and the female reproductive cycle. In addition, this peaceful luminary is the heavenly body that governs the astrological sign of Cancer, which is in turn the sign of home and mother. In both yoga and Oriental Medicine (OM), the moon is associated with female energy, called ida *and* yin *respectively in these traditions.*

Pulling Down the Moon

The idea of "pulling down the moon" calls to mind the challenges that many of us face when trying to conceive. It is during this time that our femininity feels challenged, that some of us may feel that motherhood is as far away as the moon and just as hard to reach. Yet, we all have exactly what we need to be happy and complete, and it is often the self-realization of this fact that is the challenge. Tami and Beth had both experienced their fertility journey and motherhood as a call to self-realization and wanted to pass this experience along.

And so they found their name and their mission. When they offered their first class in Chicago, they called it Pulling Down the Moon, and a year later when they opened their first center, that's what they called it, too. And it was everything they'd hoped it would be. Since they began, they have brought on many loving practitioners, like Jeanie Lee Bussell, who have helped to deepen the understanding of how the healing arts can impact fertility. The Fully Fertile program is a distillation of practices we have developed over the years at Pulling Down the Moon. We hope you will find peace, healing, and fertility in the pages that follow.

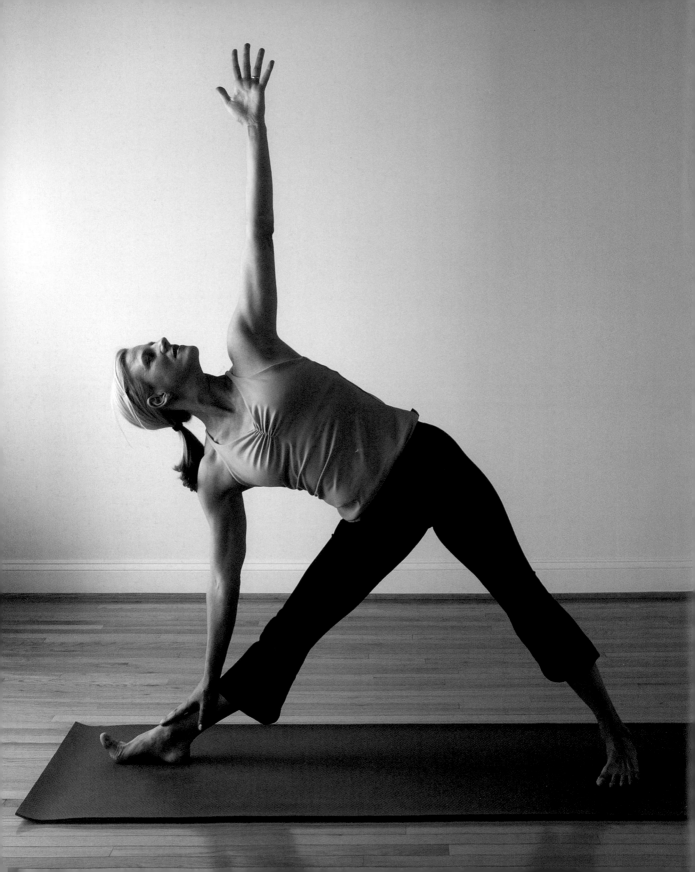

How to Use this Book

Tapa Swadhaya Ishwara Pranidhani Kriya Yogah
Yoga Sutras of Patanjali, II, 1

FULLY FERTILE is set up for use as a twelve-week program to optimize fertility. The sequence of the program is not random. It is based on two ancient teachings from yoga philosophy that outline practical methods for attaining unshakable peace and happiness, or "yoga." These practices, while macrocosmic in origin, can be brought to bear on more specific life challenges, such as fertility. In this way, the entire Fully Fertile program is contained within a context that is designed to imbue even the most basic choices, such as what foods we choose to eat or how we move our body, with the power of spirit and sacred intention. We feel this is why women who come to us in search of family often leave us with more than just babies. By working with these profound concepts they also gain greater self-love and inner peace. Yoga is, after all, the process of reuniting with Self, and finding peace and contentment in the process.

Yoga of Action

The first yoga concept, which has guided the division of this book into its structure of three separate phases, focusing on the physical, mental, and spiritual aspects of the fertility journey respectively, arises from the second chapter of the *Yoga Sutras* which were written by the sage Patanjali around 200 BCE. In this chapter, Patanjali describes a three-part method of attaining yoga (union with Self). Patanjali's method includes *tapas* (purification), *svadyaya* (self-study) and *ishvara pranhidana* (surrender to the divine). This path, says Patanjali, is particularly useful for those of us who are not as good at "letting go and letting God" and who feel compelled to take action in our search for happiness. Because it is good for us "do-er types," this method is also called the path of *kriya* yoga, or the yoga of action. The word tapas comes from the word tapa, meaning to burn. Practices of tapas include creating a healthy discipline of diet, exercise, abstention from toxic behaviors, and a "burning desire to achieve purification." Phase One of the Fully Fertile program is devoted entirely to the tapas of fertility—making changes to our exercise, to our diet, to the quality of our sleep and sex lives. In this chapter we seek to use our motivation to become pregnant to help us purify our physical being. The second phase of the book will take us beyond the physical practice of tapas into the practice of svadyaya, or self-study. In this section of the book we will work on letting go of the expectations, judgments and negative thoughts we have created around the fertility journey and our own, innate fertility. In this section you will be challenged to dredge up your mental garbage and "read" the fertility story you've written for yourself with a critical eye. Finally, in Phase Three, the shift is made to Spirit. Ishvara pranhidana means "surrender to the Divine." In this section we will explore some of the more esoteric tools of yoga, including breathing, meditation, and prayer, which can create powerful shifts in our fertility journey if we open to them.

The Kosha Model

The second concept that guides our programming at Pulling Down the Moon as well as informs this book is the *kosha* model. This model for yoga healing was first outlined in the

The Five Koshas

1. The Physical Body (Annamaya Kosha) *includes our flesh, bone, skin, and organs. For the purpose of this book, you will work with the Physical Body through yoga practice, Oriental Medicine, fertility nutrition, and healthy sleep and sex.*

2. The Energy Body (Pranamaya Kosha) *includes life energy (prana/chi) and the system of energy circulation; breathing, nadis/meridians. Throughout this book you will be nourishing your Energy Body with specific yoga and Oriental Medicine breathing techniques.*

3. The Psycho-Emotional Body (Manomaya Kosha) *includes all aspects of everyday thought and emotion, including our stressors, dealing with disappointment and overall attitudes toward our fertility.*

4. The Wisdom Body (Vijnanamaya Kosha) *is our intellect and our intuition, two facilities that allow us to see the forest for the trees. Healing in the Wisdom Body comes through self-study as well as the company of others who are seeking similar truth, and the reading and study of sacred scriptures and meditation.*

5. The Bliss Body (Anandamaya Kosha) *is a deep appreciation of life that arises from connection with the part of ourselves that is not apart from the universal Self. Knowledge and the healing of the bliss body comes from surrender and devotion to God (ishvara pranidhana), or simply through the practice of happiness and gratitude.*

Upanishads, a collection of oral teachings transmitted from guru to disciple many thousands of years ago. Way ahead of its time, the kosha model asserts that we have more than just one body; in fact we have five bodies, called koshas.

Yoga therapy teaches that an illness can arise from separation at the level of one or more of the koshas. The first tool in healing is awareness. This awareness comes from the mental and physical connection you make that something is out of balance. As you work to integrate body, mind, and spirit, the healing process can be spontaneous.

Integrative Care for Fertility

When we teach these concepts to our students in yoga class we call them by their Sanskrit names. When we speak to healthcare providers, we call our approach Integrative Care for Fertility, or ICF™. It is a holistic way of enhancing fertility, and it has received a warm reception from those in the medical fertility community, who are becoming increasingly alarmed at the high rates of stress and anxiety they see in their patients. Because medical practices are focused on providing the best medical fertility treatment available, there's often insufficient time for a physician to devote to helping us do the kinds of things that need to be done outside the walls of their practice to make us fully fertile. If you're not working with a physician on your road to having a child, ICF can help you as well. These steps will help anyone create a happier, healthier, more fully fertile body.

The Fully Fertile Program

So now that you know that the Fully Fertile program was created to help you access the gifts of kriya yoga and the healing model of the koshas, how do you use this book? We suggest the following guidelines:

• Read the book start to finish before starting the program.
• Get a pretty journal or notebook to hold your nutrition log, your sleep/dream journal, as well as the answers to the exercises you will be given over the course of twelve weeks. A companion notebook to this book is available at *www.pullingdownthemoon.com*.
• Where possible, create sangha. Sangha is a group of like-minded people sharing a similar intention. If you know another woman who is also having difficulty conceiving, invite her to do the program with you. You will benefit from the motivation of having a yoga buddy, going grocery shopping together, and sharing recipes, as well as discussing some of the exercises in Phases 2 and 3.
• Consider starting a Fully Fertile group. Contact Pulling Down the Moon and we can connect you with others in your area who are working with this program.
• You can also visit *www.pullingdownthemoon.com* for supplies, products, and support.

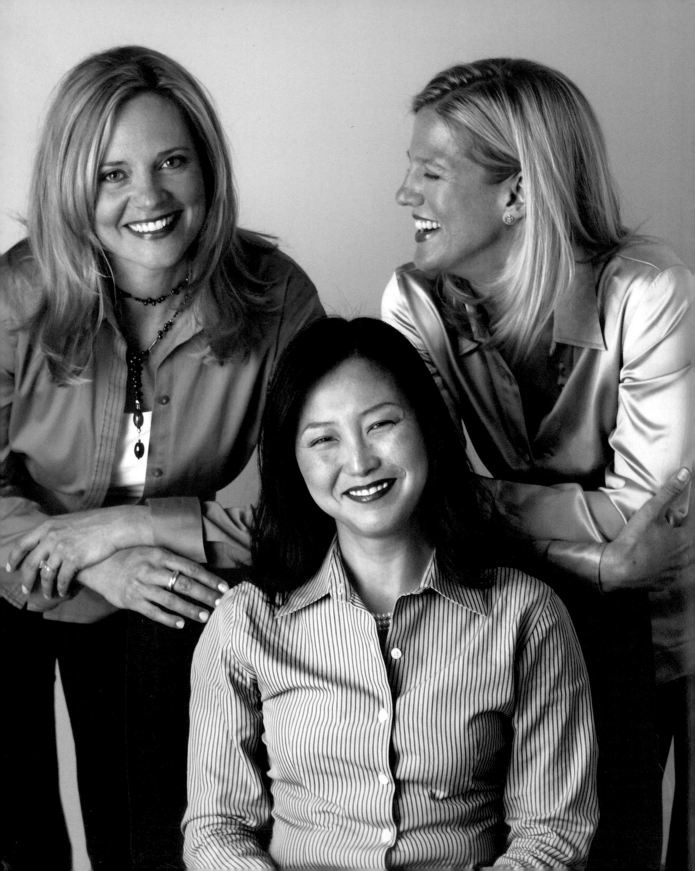

Our Stories

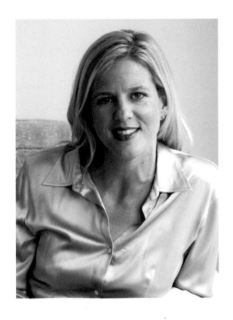

BETH'S STORY

AS I SIT HERE, typing with one hand and feeding a scrambled egg to my little one with the other, it feels like I am literally writing the last chapter of my fertility journey. Jackson, my oldest, is now three and a half and Calvin will be one next week. The mundane events that have punctuated the writing of this book—much of which has been written between endless games of Candyland with Jackson and to the beat of Calvin's hands on the tray of his highchair—still give me pause for deepest gratitude. It was a long road to find these guys—seven years from when I started to Calvin's arrival.

Like many women, my attitude toward parenting went from "some day" to "I want to be pregnant yesterday" surprisingly quickly. When the idea of being a parent first began to shift from the distant, hazy future to something nearer and more concrete, I was a stressed-out graduate student, working toward a PhD in nutrition, and up to my neck in a National Institute of Health research study examining the impact of walking on the physical and emotional well-being of menopausal women.

Looking back, I see the roots of the holistic outlook developed at Pulling Down the Moon coming from this period. At the time, our research group was among the first to question the blanket prescription of estrogen replacement therapy for the treatment of menopausal symptoms. Measuring how much something as simple as a walking program and group support could impact women's depression and anxiety rates, their overall health and their perception of themselves as "strong and vital" versus "getting old" would eventually shape my attitudes about my own and others' fertility issues. Unfortunately, at the time it just added up to a ton of work, deadlines, papers, exams, and a job doing personal training on the side to supplement my research stipend. Add to that an addiction to running that made me clock upward of thirty miles per week; basically, I was spent.

Nevertheless, I started to think about pregnancy. I'd been married for seven years at that point and my husband Matt and I had discussed having kids but didn't really have a schedule. It was more like "we'll have them when we're ready"—as if life would put a note on our Yahoo! Calendar that it was time to get started on a family. Finally, because it seemed like a good place to start, I stopped taking the Pill. Even that was a big drama. I lectured Matt on the need for other methods of birth control, because even though I'd stopped the Pill, I wasn't quite ready to be a mom yet.

So, we stopped the Pill and prepared to have to try not to get pregnant for a while. That proved to be pretty laughable. A few months post-Pill my periods were still conspicuously absent. Nevertheless, the high-school health class mentality of "you can get pregnant from a toilet seat" was firmly ingrained in my mind. Even without my period, I was sure I would still get pregnant, so we kept using those condoms. Technically, I could get pregnant. But only if I was ovulating, which I definitely was not.

Anyhow, I wasn't in a big rush. I had my graduate work to finish and the biological clock had not yet reached panic decibel. I was busy collecting data, writing papers and struggling to keep my head above water in the stressful world of academia. When my amenorrhea (lack of menstruation) stretched well into its third year, I finally consulted an endocrine specialist at a local, well-respected hospital. I was relieved to find he wasn't particularly concerned. I was not so relieved when he pronounced that I was a "classic case of hypothalamic amenorrhea" and invited all five of the medical residents he had in tow to do a pelvic exam on me. Remember that this was in the years before my fertility travels, when I wasn't the old pro I am now with the vaginal ultrasounds and the stirrups.

"There are medical interventions we can use when you're really ready to have a baby," the doctor said when we sat down to discuss my situation.

That was the sum total of his advice. Call me crazy, but I thought there'd be more. He made no effort to ask any simple lifestyle questions to see why I was amenorrheic, and certainly had no suggestions or strategies to help me restore my menses. I left his office feeling like my only option was to remain amenorrheic until I decided to take fertility medication. To be honest, it really rubbed me the wrong way. Especially when my own subsequent research revealed "hypothalamic amenorrhea" could result from a wide range of lifestyle conditions including stress, anxiety, depression, eating disorders, and poor sleep—of which many are common in the modern graduate student.

Not long after that doctor visit, I woke up one morning to find that the baby bug had bit me overnight. The endocrinologist's promise of "the things we could do when I was ready" echoed in my brain. For better or for worse, though, the stubborn, holistic side of me that had spent three years teaching menopausal women how to improve their health and quality of life with a walking program suddenly spoke up. I knew the doctor had things he could do, but there were also things I could do on my own. If hypothalamic amenorrhea really was associated with stress and fatigue, I knew two places I could start.

It was about the time that I heard the infamous Voice that told me to stop what I was doing and make some changes (you will read more about this wacko experience at the beginning of Phase 1 of this book). Listening to that Voice—who can argue with a Voice?— I wandered into my first yoga class exhausted and frazzled and walked out feeling nourished and centered. It was that simple for me. That very day I bought a book, a mat, and started to create a yoga practice that I would do almost every day. The second thing I did was start to talk to a psychotherapist about learning to slow down. Amazingly, about three months after starting my yoga practice and therapy, my period returned after a four-year absence.

Taking a Holistic Route

Of course I thought I had the whole fertility thing figured out. And my belief was confirmed when, a few months after that first cycle, I got pregnant! When I told my husband the news, we both laughed at how easy it had turned out to be after all!

"It's elementary, Watson. Just do yoga!"

Not so fast, Holmes. A few weeks later I had a miscarriage.

Certainly it was a devastating event, and one that I speak about later on in the book. Yet, I was still deep in the throes of my early romance with yoga and pretty sure that I was on the right track. When I started "trying" again I got right down to brass tacks. I charted my BBT, made changes to my diet on the advice of an Ayurvedic physician, took herbs, and, of course, kept doing my yoga. It was like I didn't really realize how badly I wanted a baby until I had that miscarriage. Still, I was only 32 and felt committed to a holistic route to pregnancy.

During the time that I was "trying," I entered yoga teacher training, dropped out of my PhD program and finished with a Master's Degree, and became a full-time yoga instructor. As part of my yoga training I wrote a thesis on using yoga to help fertility. Sometimes I wonder what kept me on the holistic path during those months. My obstetrician (OB) was wonderfully supportive, even apologizing before she gently suggested I could try Clomid (see p. 73), but I declined. Although it was challenging at times, with disappointment each time another month passed without pregnancy, it was also a time of profound learning. As I was charting my cycles I learned that my luteal phase was short—something that led me to research vitamin supplementation, the nutritional impact of oral contraceptives and the effect of exercise on the menstrual cycle. And the coolest part was watching my cycles get stronger and my luteal phase lengthen. In addition, I began to witness profound shifts in my own life. I felt stronger, healthier, and more grounded than I ever had in my life. My schedule and lifestyle were saner, my diet healthier and more nurturing than ever before.

I finally conceived again in November 2002, fifteen months after the miscarriage. Once I got past the panic of the first trimester, it was a smooth-sailing time. I felt great, the baby was growing, and I absolutely loved being pregnant. Before we found out I was pregnant we had planned to take a trip to Europe in what would be the seventh month of pregnancy. With our OB's blessing we took the trip and had an amazing time. There's a picture that my husband took that crystallizes this time in my life. He snapped it on a gorgeous afternoon in Switzerland when we were walking in the high Alps. I'm just a tiny speck, but an obviously pregnant one, on a path with enormous, gorgeous alpine mountains behind me. It's sunny and you can just feel my happiness. I was talking to my baby that day as I walked, telling him or her how I had met their daddy in France and that our first "date" had been a weekend trip right here in Switzerland. I was lost in pregnant day-dreams about a return trip, with a tiny baby in a backpack. Dreams of pure joy…

Pulling Down the Moon

Three weeks after we returned home from Europe my friends had a baby shower for me. I got absolutely everything I could possibly need for this baby. Clothes, strollers, a bassinet, blankets… but sadly, I wouldn't need any of it. A week after the shower our baby was still-born. It was a fluke thing, a cord incident that caused the baby, a little girl that we named Georgia, to lose access to oxygen and die. She was absolutely perfect in every other way— and a very special person in my life in ways that I would only later learn.

So how do you pick up the pieces? In my case (no surprise), I did yoga. Despite the absolute horror and disappointment of Georgia's stillbirth, her arrival marked a fundamental shift in my life. I went from thinking I had things pretty much figured out to knowing that our sense of control over the fragility of life is an illusion. Certainly, we can and should do everything possible to live a healthy life, to keep ourselves and our loved ones safe…but ultimately there's an element of mystery at play in determining the outcomes of our hopes and dreams. Yoga, with its emphasis on each breath, on the beauty of each moment, of letting go of emotions that cloud our perception of the present, was an amazing way to heal from this devastating experience. I also had the help of many loving friends, amazing parents and in-laws, and a husband who accepted this experience in the same light that I did, as part of the larger spiritual practice called life. Another shift occurred as well. Having come so close to having a baby I was now sure that it didn't matter how I was going to get the next one. Losing Georgia made one thing crystal clear to me: biological, adopted, or cabbage patch, I just wanted a baby. I opened whole-heartedly to the universe—praying that a child, any child, would find its way to me and Matt.

Shortly after Georgia died, I met Tami Quinn and we started our first fertility yoga class, calling it "Pulling Down the Moon." At first, when I would teach, I would cry each time I told my Georgia story. We used to joke that it was the story that could crack even the toughest nut in the house. Not long after starting the class, I returned to the work of getting pregnant again. This time it was not bliss. It was a hurdle—and one that terrified me.

First off, I wanted fertility drugs and I wanted them now. Luckily (and I believe largely thanks to yoga, a fertility-friendly diet, and other holistic practices), I conceived on my fifth cycle of Clomid. The first trimester was hell (I will be eternally grateful to the ultrasonographer at my reproductive endocrinologist's office who snuck me in for extra "heartbeat" checks whenever I showed up at her door in the midst of a panic attack). But miracle of miracles, the baby's heart kept beating and after nine of the longest months *ever* I gave birth to a healthy baby boy, Jackson George Heller.

Needless to say, it was an amazing day.

About a year and a half after Jackson was born, it was time to go back into the trying-to-conceive trenches. We really wanted a sibling for Georgia and Jack. Even though I had continued with my yoga and my holistic approach to life, I was geared up for a struggle and perhaps even the need for more intensive fertility treatments because now I was 37 years old with a *history* of infertility. And then an amazing thing happened. One month after I started acupuncture and herbs for fertility I conceived naturally *the first time we tried*. Now I know this doesn't happen in every case, but it again bolstered my belief that we can improve our fertility by cultivating a life of balance. Nine months later, Calvin was born hale and hearty and the journey was drawing to a close.

Full Circle to Fully Fertile

Each subsequent day with Jackson, and now Calvin, has been an amazing adventure and a blessing. When Jackson arrived and I finally was holding my baby, a weight was undoubtedly lifted from my heart. Yet I also recognized a fundamental truth. The stress, sorrow, and anxiety associated with my infertility and losses did not disappear; they simply changed focus. Now my worries became Jackson's health, my growing business, and the changing nature of my relationship with my husband as we learned to become parents after 13 years of marriage. And once again, I was drawn back to practice. Yoga, for all the reasons I've already mentioned, provided my framework for coping with the new challenges of motherhood and life as an entrepreneur. The work I had done in preparing for Jackson was essential training for motherhood and beyond.

I still tell Georgia's story at the start of every class, but time has healed much of the pain and my eyes are dry when I talk about these experiences. There continue to be amazing coincidences over the years that make me feel that her spirit is nearby. Shortly after we opened our first Pulling Down the Moon in Chicago, I walked into the tearoom to find a single sticky name tag with "Georgia" written on it. When I asked our staff if we had a Georgia in for class or for treatment they were baffled. No Georgia had come through the door. Some would call it coincidence, but I choose to think she was saying hello. There's no question in my mind that she approves of the work we do at Pulling Down the Moon. Sometimes I think it's why she entered my life in the first place—to give me the courage to help other women who were struggling to become mothers.

But ghost stories aside, Georgia's gift to me is the knowledge that my identity as a mother was not dependent on having a child. As I went on with Tami Quinn to teach fertility yoga and to open Pulling Down the Moon, I was able to speak with the conviction that true fertility is within us and comes when we recognize our self-worth and our innate ability to nurture and sustain others. Now, as I write those words, tears come again to my eyes. I have come full circle and I have chills because I know Georgia's here with me as I write. At Pulling Down the Moon, we believe that each woman will eventually find the child she's meant to have, even if the child doesn't arrive in the way or in the timeframe that she planned or expected it to. Even with all the amazing technological and holistic treatments described in this book, some women will need to adopt, or use donor gametes or a gestational surrogate in order to find that baby. But if she can open her heart to any possibility of parenting and above all learn to love herself, she will truly be fully fertile.

JEANIE'S STORY

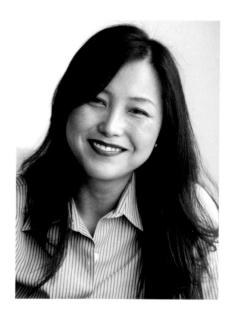

I GREW UP in a culture where herbs and acupuncture had long been the primary care of the people. As long as I remember, I wanted to be an acupuncturist and herbalist. For me, my grandmother was the primary care "doctor," whose hands and knowledge treated everything from the common cold to menstrual difficulties. Getting acupuncture for stomach aches and taking herbal decoctions for colds and coughs were commonplace in my household. Our diet and herbal teas varied with each season to "supplement" our bodies to withstand the changes of the environment. In the summer we ate cooling foods; and in the winter, we ate warming foods (this sounds like common sense but it's not what is practiced in most of America). As most women know, periods start to sync with one another when you live with other women. With three girls and mom in our family, our periods synced with each other all the time. Just imagine four women having their period in a house of six! At the end of each period, my grandmother got busy with our diet and herbal teas to "replenish" the lost "heavenly Blood." We were told not to sit on cold surfaces, or play or do anything strenuous, for it would hurt our Qi (life energy) during our menstruation. We were told to take grandmother's advice seriously because, according to her, not replenishing period blood properly, sitting on cold surfaces, and engaging in strenuous activities (such as playing sports) during menstruation would have an effect on our future fertility. I remember my grandmother saying every time I sat on the metal steps on our back porch that the cold energy of the metal steps would "freeze" my reproductive area and that would hurt my ability to have children when I got older. Every time I thought, "there she goes again with her old superstition." Now that I am a practitioner of Oriental Medicine, I now understand and honor her wisdom and knowledge in what I once believed to be "old superstition."

After studying biology at the University of Maryland, I moved to Chicago to pursue study in pharmacy. Not knowing that there are programs in Oriental Medicine in the United States, I thought pharmacy was the closest thing to "herbology." Fortunately, Chicago was home to one of the oldest Oriental Medicine schools in the country. Without hesitation, I switched my career path and enrolled at Midwest College of Oriental Medicine. It was there that I met my future husband Jason.

Finding My Path

Toward the end of my years at Midwest College, I went to China to take advanced courses and participate in a clinical internship in the state hospitals. It was an amazing experience which taught me a lot, but it was also very demanding and stressful. I had an incident of abnormal uterine bleeding shortly after I returned. At first I thought it was stress and ignored the symptom. But it did not stop and after three days of continual bleeding, I started to have abdominal cramps. That's when I took myself to the hospital to find that I had an ovarian tumor on my right side that was about the size of a large orange. My doctor recommended surgery, but since it was benign, she agreed to let me try Oriental Medicine first. After three months of regular acupuncture treatments, herbal therapy, meditation, and Qi Gong, I went back for my follow-up ultrasound. I am sure most of you who are reading this know that trans-vaginal ultrasounds are not the most pleasant experience. I think I had one of the most painful trans-vaginal ultrasounds of my life that day! The ultrasound technologist was looking for the tumor but it was not showing up on the ultrasound. Needless to say my ultrasound report stated "inconclusive" and I was ordered for a CT scan. The CT report came back reading "unremarkable." This demonstrated to me the power of Oriental Medicine and ignited my passion for working with women's health. My master's thesis was on the most important herbal prescriptions for American female patients.

After graduation, my husband and I opened up a private practice in a suburb of Chicago. It quickly became apparent that fertility was a great concern for many women. A colleague and I began devising a research proposal to investigate acupuncture's ability to help improve fertility. That's when I met Beth Heller, one of the co-founders of Pulling Down the Moon, at a local yoga studio.

Looking very pregnant, Beth told me that she and her business partner, Tami Quinn, had heard about me and had meant to come and visit me at my office. She told me about their intention to open an integrative center for fertility and asked if I knew much about fertility acupuncture. Since I had specialized in women's health and was currently working on a similar project, I was familiar with the research that had been published and the techniques that were used. I did not have much experience with treating fertility at that point, but Tami and Beth took a chance on me.

My first few months of treating fertility at Pulling Down the Moon were very difficult. No one got pregnant! It tore me up because I got so attached to my patients and their dreams. Each negative pregnancy test felt like a huge failure on my part. A famous Oriental Medical gynecologist, Bob Flaws, explained it well when he said why he no longer treats fertility. There is no partial success. With acupuncture, if you come in with severe pain and the acupuncture knocks it down to moderate pain, we can both be pretty happy about that. But with fertility, even if I help women develop more and healthier eggs, the ideal endometrium, balanced hormones, and help to promote implantation, if it does not result in a live birth, it is all for naught. My lack of success early on was very difficult for me and I considered giving up treating fertility patients.

Instead, I poured myself into my study. I bought and read every book on the subject. I traveled around the country and Asia to study with the masters in this field. I felt a compulsion to become the best I could be. Although I would never have chosen this disappointment for myself or for my patients, it forced me to become a better practitioner and student.

After some time with Pulling Down the Moon, Tami and Beth named me as Director of Acupuncture for the three centers. I was in charge of hiring and training all the acupuncturists. Again I felt pressure to be the best. Now even more couples and other practitioners were depending on my expertise. This forced me to study even harder. Looking back, these challenges may have been the best things that could have happened to me and my practice. I still attend seminars on the topic, but now I also present them and teach my peers how to understand and treat this complex problem.

In my years with Pulling Down the Moon, I have treated thousands of women for fertility and feel very comfortable doing it. It can still be very draining emotionally but it can also be very rewarding. At our office, we have pictures of babies of women who were told that they could never conceive their own child. People ask how long the effects of acupuncture last and I answer, "Maybe a hundred years." I feel blessed to be able to use this huge body of knowledge that is Oriental Medicine to help couples realize one of their most important desires—the desire to have a family.

TAMI'S STORY

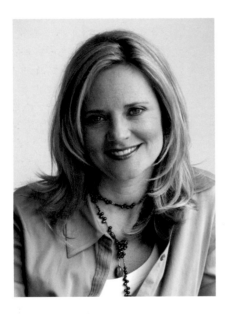

I MARRIED BRIAN when I was 26 years old. He knew when he married me that I had a penchant for the mystical. I enjoyed astrology, read a lot of books about self-healing, practiced meditation, and joked with him that I was psychic and knew exactly what he was thinking. Too bad I wasn't psychic enough to predict that my journey to motherhood and my path to yoga would be paved with challenges before arriving at my final destination.

When we got engaged, I told Brian I didn't want to entertain the idea of having children until I was at least 30 years old. I needed to "experience the world" and figured we should have four or five years to travel, work our way up the corporate ladder, put away our nest egg, and stay out late without the worry of children.

Shortly after we married I landed my dream job in advertising at a brand new magazine called *Martha Stewart Living*. I worked hard those years because I truly liked my job, loved the magazine, the lifestyle it represented, and the fat paycheck that reflected my strong effort on the job.

We bought and renovated a house near Wrigley Field in Chicago about a year later and then subsequently took a two-week trip to Italy. Our first five years of marriage had been great. We did exactly what I had wanted to do: traveled, went antiquing, changed jobs, bought our dream house, and spent every Thursday night in front of the TV after work watching *Friends, Seinfeld,* and *ER.* Life was good and I felt I had checked everything off my "to do" list, so I announced to Brian that the time had come to go off the Pill. One of my best girlfriends had already had a baby and many were beginning to try. Yes, they were getting bit by the baby bug and I certainly did not want to be left behind. When my friend Barbara had her son William, I went to visit her in the hospital and held a newborn for the very first time. I watched her nurse and coddle him and something magical happened inside of me. It's one thing to talk about having a child, to think about it in some abstract, futuristic way. It's another thing to actually hold a baby in your arms and experience the miracle that is creation, the bond that is mother and child. I was sold! No more thinking or waiting, I wanted a baby now.

Although other good friends like Karen and Chrissy had been going through some infertility issues, I was convinced I'd have no problem. After all, I was a healthy "type A" over-achiever whose parents always taught her that if you work hard enough, you will usually attain your goals. Since I had accomplished nearly every other goal I had set in my life, I figured baby-making would be no different. Besides, Sister Joan of Arc, one of my teachers in junior high, always said, "It just takes one time."

When it didn't happen within the first three months I was a bit surprised and decided I must not have been taking the task seriously enough. I went out and bought a handful of books about getting pregnant, made an appointment with my OB, had my blood analyzed, bought some prenatal vitamins, began researching fertility, and went back to the bedroom. Mind you, this was before there were websites and chat boards about getting pregnant. With so many changes and advances in medical fertility, by the time I found and read articles or books at the library, the information was nearly obsolete.

Chasing the Dream

When I still wasn't getting pregnant, I decided to start tracking my basal body temperature to ensure we were hitting my exact day of ovulation. It became an obsession. I had graph paper, colored pencils, and thermometers all lined up next to my bed. I wouldn't even lift my head off the pillow without taking my temperature for fear of getting an inaccurate reading. God forbid I should have to go to the bathroom or answer a phone call in the early morning hours for fear of foiling a whole day's worth of temperatures. After four months of this, I reported back to my OB with graphs in hand. He took one look and announced that I was not ovulating and would probably need Clomid to increase my chances of releasing an egg. I was so excited to get the meds I nearly skipped home. It meant pregnancy was not too far off. Plus I knew it increased my chances of having multiples, which I had decided (at the age of ten) would be a very efficient way of family building. Three cycles later, however, I still was not pregnant. I went back to the OB and he added a shot of hCG to my protocol, which not only upped my hormone levels but my mood swings, too. Much to my own surprise, I conceived that month and made a happy transition from the "How to Get Pregnant" books to the "You *are* Pregnant" books. Sadly, I miscarried in my sixth week while making sales calls in St. Louis.

Miscarrying is so terribly difficult; it doesn't matter how far along you are in a pregnancy. Even though the idea of a child was only six weeks old in my mind, my body had already begun to change. My breasts were tender and my belly felt slightly full. Emotionally, I had already prepared for his/her arrival by marking the due date on a calendar. When I erased that entry in my day planner I remember it was like wiping away a dream that was beginning to elude me.

A bit broken-hearted and growing increasingly worried, I returned to my OB who now prescribed Intra-uterine Inseminations (IUI). Despite additional medications, increased monitoring, a cooperative husband, and fancy chairs that tipped me nearly upside down, I was not getting pregnant so I asked my doctor to refer me to a reproductive endocrinologist (RE). Every time I got a new medical protocol I felt lighthearted, optimistic, and hopeful again. I convinced myself that this time it would work.

While under the care of the reproductive endocrinologist, I went for a series of tests like the hysterosalpingogram (HSG) and then began taking injectable medications to help stimulate egg production and, hopefully, end this problem of being anovulatory. My hope turned to despair after the first failed cycle. I remember walking back from the RE's office with my husband and lamenting to him that this might never happen. He was much more optimistic than I and said, "If we want to be parents, we will be parents." He had given me permission to fail. He had forced me to think a thought I had never thought before. What was more important to me? Being a parent or having a biological child? For me, the answer was clear. I wanted a child and if that meant using a donor or adopting a baby, I could be okay with that. Ironically, the following month I conceived twins, a boy and a girl (Kevin and Courtney), who were born healthy and happy nine months later.

After my struggles with getting pregnant and then carrying and delivering twins, I vowed I would never forget about how challenging and isolating the process was. I thought, perhaps, one day I would write a book about conceiving and carrying multiples that would provide other women with the support I lacked on my journey. What I didn't realize, though, was that the book would not be written in the way I had imagined because my challenges were just beginning. The book needed to have another experiential life chapter.

My twins were not good sleepers and when they were up in the middle of the night, it meant that two parents had to be up feeding them. Brian and I got very little sleep the first two years of Courtney and Kevin's lives. Let me tell you, I now understand how sleep deprivation could have been used as a form of torture against POWs during World War II. It's okay for a week or two, but after two years you can't even think straight. Added to the difficulty of sleepless nights, my job at *Martha Stewart Living* became increasingly more difficult and stressful. I had a new boss in New York who operated on a 24/7 schedule that meant that I was literally on call all the time. I was fielding phone calls in the evenings and on Sunday afternoons on top of the hours already spent in the office. It was all business all of the time. Although I eliminated much of my overnight travel, I was still doing a lot of day trips, which were mentally and physically exhausting. My full-time nanny gave me the confidence to know that the kids were being well cared for, but I still felt like I was living in two different worlds and not really doing anything very well. I was not completely entrenched in the mom world and not really 100 percent in the career world. There was just not enough time in the day for me to fulfill all of my obligations and I hated feeling like I was doing things half way.

We sold our home in the city and bought a house in the suburbs with a big back yard for the kids to play in. It required extensive remodeling, so Brian and I added that to our plate. My life was now busier than I could handle and I found myself torn between wanting to be home all the time with my kids and wanting to have a career. Beyond the intellectual stimulation, my job provided a paycheck that was now a necessity, as we had a new house to pay for. My kids were three and I still felt stuck, wishing someone would just wave a magic wand and tell me what to do with my life or make me drink the magic potion that would allow me to "have it all."

Martha Stewart had just taken her company public and that meant lucrative stock options for those founding employees who would stick around long enough to be vested in the company. Great, I now had the paradoxical golden handcuffs keeping me tied to the corporate world.

Yoga for Life

During my drive home from work and at the park when I watched the kids play, I began to contemplate some existential questions: If I'm not a career woman, what am I? Would it be enough for me to just be a mom and a housewife? Was that spicy enough chit chat for my neighborhood cocktail parties? Could we really afford my quitting? Struggling with these questions made me increasingly anxious. My biggest joy was being with my children but financially I was fearful that I couldn't afford to be with them all the time.

One morning, I was reading through my community recreation center bulletin and noticed there were yoga classes being offered. Although yoga was not the hot bed of popularity it is now, I had heard some anecdotal stories that yoga was good for stress, so I decided to sign up for a class. When I first started doing yoga, I kept my cell phone on vibrate and would leave the room to answer business calls and urgent messages from the nanny. My mind would race a million thoughts a minute and I found it extremely difficult to focus or "be still," as the yoga teacher instructed. I stuck with it anyway. The more I did yoga the better I felt physically and mentally and the more clarity I had. As I started realizing it was helping in these ways, I became hungrier for deeper meaning behind the ancient spiritual science of yoga. I started delving into spiritual texts, attended lectures, and ate up the esoteric tools I found hidden underneath the yoga postures. It was more than just exercise; it was an entire handbook on how to live life, and the more I copied instruction from this mystical manual the more my life began to change for the better. I decided to quit my job, be a stay-at-home mom, and started taking yoga philosophy classes through the Temple of Kriya in Chicago. At the Temple, I met my guru, Goswami Kriyananda, who guided me through advanced teachings on meditation, breathing, religions of the world, astrology, dream symbols, mantra, and self-realization. I did not know where the path would lead, but I knew in my heart that it would be revealed, and vowed to somehow share these healing techniques with others when the time came. I eventually became an ordained swami as a symbol of commitment to this promise.

Kriyananda taught me that the tools and techniques passed down through thousands of years of tradition are practices that allow the seeker to live a happier, healthier, and more meaningful life. I knew from experience these tools worked and then, one day, I was approached by my kids' kindergarten teacher, who asked if yoga could help fertility. I knew then and there that this would be my calling. I knew that yoga could be invaluable for women trying to conceive because it worked on all aspects of a person: her mind, body, and spirit. That's what I needed when I was challenged with infertility and I knew that's what other women would need too. With that in mind, Beth Heller and I started Pulling Down the Moon one year after I quit my job at *Martha Stewart Living*. Today I am still living in the world as both a mother and businesswoman, but now life is on my terms. Pulling Down the Moon has been a blessing on so many levels. First, it is a job that allows me to control my hours so I am able to spend more time with my children and, secondly, it has given me the opportunity to combine my love of yoga with helping a population of women with whom I can relate. So, for now, the dark days of my life have left and the light has returned like the solstice in December. I'm not going to kid myself into thinking there won't be more challenges and chapters to write in the book of life but, for now, I feel yoga has given me the armor to feel well-prepared for the battle.

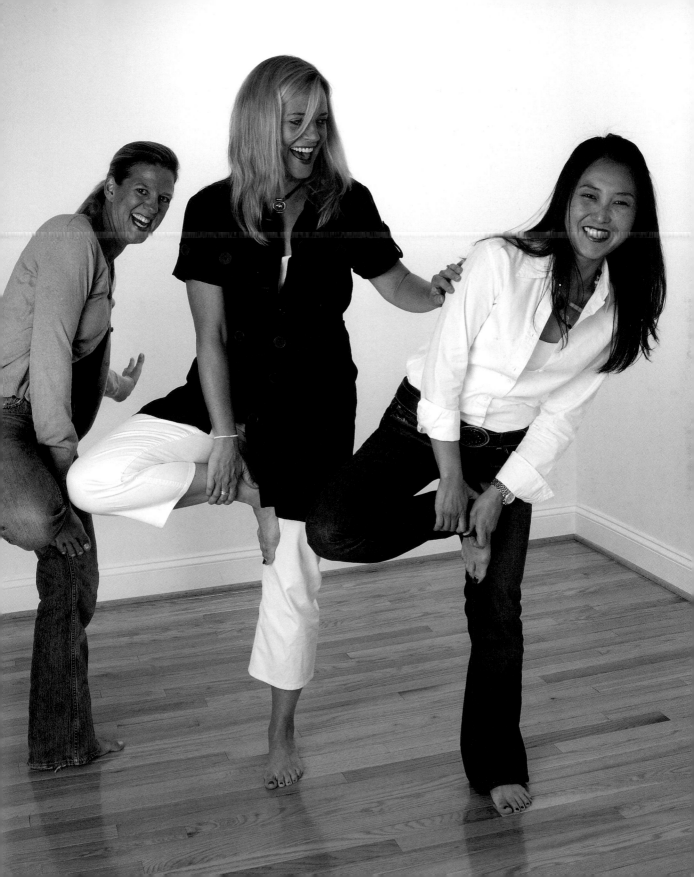

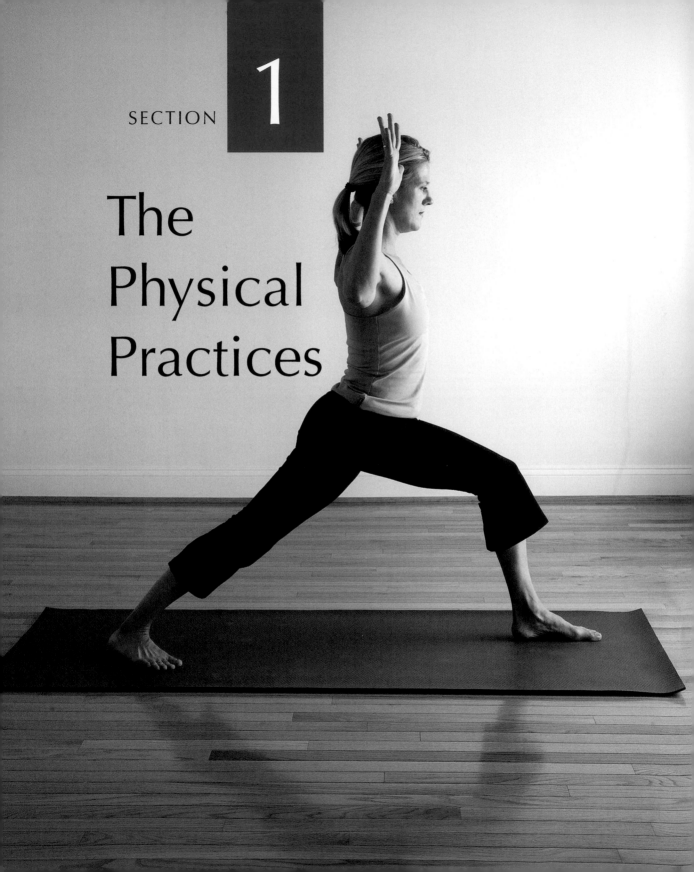

SECTION

1

The Physical Practices

Yoga Program for Fertility

Beth writes:

I can remember the day that I started my fertility journey like it was yesterday. I was in graduate school for a doctorate in nutrition at the time, working as an investigator on a big NIH-funded grant, seeing clients part-time as a personal trainer at my local gym, and working my body pretty hard as a runner.

I had been amenorrheic (no periods) since I stopped taking my birth control pills four years previously. The fact that my periods had not returned didn't seem to concern anybody too much. I was only 30, my body weight and body fat were both normal. I worked out a lot but I wasn't bone-thin. There was a lot of stress in my life but what grad student—come to think of it, what person—didn't have stress? Nevertheless, I was beginning to get that baby itch pretty bad and, as anyone who's been there can attest, a large part of my mental capacity began to dwell on the how and when of becoming pregnant. My OB seemed confident that when I was ready to conceive I could just take Clomid to jumpstart my system.

Not long after I decided it was time to get pregnant, I was on the treadmill running my requisite five daily miles when I literally heard a voice say, "Stop." Now, I've heard voices once or twice before, but this voice spoke with an authority that was non-negotiable.

"Stop," it said again, and I did.

I hit the big red stop button on that treadmill and stumbled over my feet as the belt slowed and my heartbeats floated back down to normal. Stop. Amid the whir of the other cardio machines around me, I waited for something else.

"And what?" I asked tentatively.

There was no reply.

I was slightly irritated with the voice, whoever or whatever it was. How rude to invade my workout space. I wanted this run. I needed to exercise to control my stress, to support my ad-lib, chocolate-rich diet, and to recoup the tremendous sense of accomplishment that came with the completion of each workout. I had an hour allotted for exercise in my schedule and now it had been interrupted by a voice—a voice that wasn't offering apology or explanation. An open hour gaped ahead of me. I wandered out of the cardio area and found myself smack in front of a yoga class that was about to begin.

I'd never taken yoga before. The room was dark and quiet, and as I sat down and took off my shoes and socks I didn't yet realize the journey I was about to take. It was a journey that ultimately led to a new career, the creation of Pulling Down the Moon, my daughter and two sons. But that day in class, it was all exotic and new to me. The Sanskrit terms, the stretching and breathing, and the mindfulness with which we moved our bodies was both restorative and challenging. When we finished class with resting pose, and lay flat on our backs, surrendering the weight of our body to the universe, I was surprised to find tears running down my face.

"You're exhausted," the voice said, finally breaking its silence. "You need to rest or you're going to crash."

And it was right. I wanted to be fertile and have a child but I just felt tired and brittle and exhausted. I didn't know it then, but I was what yogis call "prana-deficient"—drained of life energy and emotionally tapped out.

I fell in love with yoga that day, walked out and bought a book and a mat, and began to teach myself how to practice, how to breathe, and how to meditate. Within three months my periods returned and within six months I was pregnant. I would shortly miscarry, but that's a story for another part of the book. Within another year I began training to teach yoga and studying the use of yoga to support and cultivate fertility.

From that first day, yoga started a process of balancing first my physical body and then my mind. Soon, I felt an intuitive urge to make changes to my diet, my exercise regimen, and my sleep habits. The clandestine cigarettes I would smoke when I crammed for exams or wrote papers suddenly felt like an affront to the balance my body was establishing. Amazingly, change was occurring organically and without struggle!

What I didn't realize at the time was that I was experiencing what I would learn was a famous phrase in yoga: "Just do the practice and all is coming."

Do the practice faithfully, with joy and with your whole heart, and don't worry so much about the results.

I now know who the voice was that spoke to me on that fateful day. It was my Self, the part of me that knows best what I need even when my little self hasn't a clue. I know because, as the years have progressed and my journey into yoga, Pulling Down the Moon, and motherhood has progressed, this voice has grown stronger and clearer.

The Fully Fertile program is, at its essence, about finding this voice and accessing your own inner wisdom. It's our physical, mental, and spiritual habits that actually block our ability to see the path. So, we will begin, just as the master teachers tell us, by doing the practice.

Yoga and Fertility

Yoga is a millenniums-old philosophical discipline that originated in what is modern-day India. The practice of yoga includes many techniques. You may be most familiar with the *asana* (postures) that are familiar to us as the yoga practiced in classes and studios. Believe it or not, this is just the tip of the yoga iceberg. The postures exist to preoccupy and heal our bodies so that our mind and spirit can move deeper into the more powerful techniques of breathing, changing our attitudes, or learning to meditate. While each of these techniques has inherent benefits and application, the overall goal of yoga is to reach a state of peace and contentment, or said differently, to achieve union with our true Selves. In this context yoga can be anything—gardening, prayer, cooking, riding horses—that helps us move ourselves to a higher vibration, or state of consciousness.

In Phase 1 our focus will be on the physical postures and breathing techniques that make up a fertility asana practice. You will learn how to breathe like a yogi and practice a series of physical yoga poses designed to detoxify and calm your body, as well as to stimulate both the endocrine and the energy systems (chakras) that support reproductive function. For maximum efficacy, this practice should be done four to five times per week over the next 12 weeks. Keep in mind the goal of your hatha yoga practice is not to be the most flexible, strongest or physically adept. Your goal is to learn to calm the body enough to be able to sit quietly for 30 uninterrupted minutes, thinking of nothing. When this becomes enjoyable, your yoga is starting to work.

Did that give you pause? We just wanted to point out that the overall goal of true yoga is not physical fitness; it is mental peace and clarity. That said, there are other signs along the way that your yoga is benefiting your fertility. Are you sleeping better? Do you feel less stressed? Is it easier for you to concentrate? Perhaps your body feels more open or you just feel better "in your own skin."

Yoga and Stress Reduction

How does yoga reduce stress? The physical practice of yoga helps to reduce stress by making us aware of the ways in which we create, store, and perpetuate stress and tension in our physical bodies. By becoming aware of patterns of stress, we ultimately can identify sources of stress and begin to eliminate behaviors and conditions in our lives that are stressful.

The primary technique in yoga for reducing stress is breathing. In the practice of yoga, the breath holds a place of honor. From a mystical standpoint, the breath is believed to bring prana, or life-energy, into the body. This life-energy is considered divine, the spark that illuminates all beings. When we are full of prana, we are healthy and at peace mentally and spiritually. For fertility, it stands to reason that we want to maximize prana. A body that is full of life energy is more hospitable to new life. In fertility yoga classes, we teach students

Prana

Prana can be drawn into the body
in various ways:
- Deep, mindful breathing
- Eating non-processed, organic foods
- Interaction with/contemplation of nature
- Prayer

Prana can also be lost or
drained through:
- Stress
- Physical illness
- Obsessive thought
- Strenuous exercise
- Poor diet, too little/too much food

to conceptualize the life energy in terms of "prana in/prana out" and to strive to create a prana surplus. Prana can be drawn in or lost in various ways. The table above lists just a few examples. We will explore prana in far more depth in the third section of this book.

The Breath

The breath is important from a Western perspective, too. Unlike other body functions, like heart rate and blood pressure, the breath is under both conscious and unconscious control. We breathe without having to think about it, but when we choose, we can speed or slow our breathing rate. In Chapter 5 we will go deeper into the science of stress. For the time being though, just recognize that stress comes with a cascade of physical symptoms (racing heart, sweating palms, and churning stomach) that seem largely out of our control. Yet if we can learn to take conscious, deep breaths in moments of stress and anxiety, we can learn to control these symptoms and breath calmly in the face of life's challenges.

Blood Flow and Toxins

Yoga poses also stretch and strengthen the physical body. We tell students that they can use asana as road maps that allow them to find the places they store stress and tension. Because many of the yoga movements are outside of our daily range of motion, it may feel as if your fertility yoga practice is leaving no stone unturned. After their first yoga class, students frequently say that they felt muscles and places in their body that they never knew existed, or hadn't felt in years. This is a good thing for several reasons.

First, one of the major reasons we believe yoga improves fertility is that it works to increase blood flow. While all physical exercise increases blood flow, some exercises direct blood primarily into the large skeletal muscles. Take running, for instance. Our blood flow increases when we go for a jog, but the major recipients of this blood are the large muscles of the legs—quadriceps, hamstrings, and calves. When we run, blood is actually shunted away from our internal organs to the muscles of movement. After a run, our muscles may actually tighten. Tight pelvic musculature can obstruct blood flow and the delivery of oxygen, nourishment, and hormones to reproductive organs, including the uterus, ovaries in women, and the testes in men. Compare this to the Hip Opener on p. 39, a seated pose that is wonderful for fertility. When we practice this posture, we are stretching the muscles of the pelvis, allowing for improved blood flow and nerve signal conductivity in the pelvic area.

In addition to increasing blood flow, asana can help us release emotional tensions and toxins that have built up over the years. One way to look at this is to imagine that your body is a sculpture that has been shaped by every experience you've ever had. The time you were hit in the nose with the softball in fourth grade is still there. So is that disaster with the cartwheel at cheerleading tryouts. The miscarriage that you've finished grieving for in your conscious life is there. As you practice different yoga poses, you may find emotions, memories, smells, and sensations are released spontaneously. We call this cellular memory. This is the notion that the cells of the living tissue that belongs to you have the ability to experience and remember everything that you do. Perhaps you've heard stories of donor organ recipients reporting newfound thoughts, memories, emotions, or personality characteristics that mirror those of their donor. The cells of our body do not easily forget. For example, if you were in a car accident that hurt your low back, you may find that intense forward folds, the point of focus of which is the low back, will bring out an emotion in your mental body relating to the accident. You may cry, be fearful, or express anger while holding that posture. Many of us will avoid the posture altogether without knowing why. We just throw our hands up and say "I just can't do it," "it hurts," or "I hate this posture!"

Satori

Another great benefit of yoga is that as you become more adept at practice, you may begin to notice imbalances in your body. At first it's just physical. One side of your neck may be tighter than the other or perhaps your yoga teacher will point out that one of your shoulders is higher than the other. You may also become conscious of the imbalance in other arenas; for example, the neckline of a new blouse may look uneven. In time you may learn to relax and release the shoulder and neck on the tight side. Days or weeks later, in class or outside of class, you may suddenly realize that your tight shoulder is your "phone shoulder," the shoulder that holds the phone as you speak with clients while typing frantic emails or preparing a report. With this realization, emotions may also follow.

"I'm always on that flipping phone. It's my job. I'm always driving and talking to my boss or some client. I totally hate my job." In yoga we would say that this tightness in the shoulder is a *satori*, or an insight we have through our asana practice on the physical and emotional level that can be applied to many aspects of our life. Negative feelings you have about your job may have manifested in the form of uneven, tight shoulders in the physical body. Anger, resentment, or other powerful emotions are invisible to the naked eye, but they act like little energy vortexes—sucking prana, or life energy, out of normal circulation.

We carry around these little bags of cellular memory for years without realizing how much they're depleting us of necessary vitality. Remember to show compassion to yourself as you experience your own satori. Your body is a sculpture that has been shaped by every experience you've ever had. Some are painful, some are sad, some are amazing and joy-filled. Yoga will reveal them all.

Not surprisingly, there's an analogous action in the physical body. In response to physical injury, emotional trauma, or chronic misalignment (the latter could be caused by something as simple as habitual bad posture) the body "splints" areas of injury or misalignment by decreasing fluid to the surrounding fascia. The resulting rigidity in the connective tissue at the injury site serves initially to protect the injury during the physical healing process, but ultimately such rigidity actually perpetuates and even exacerbates the imbalance. Previous injury and trauma in the lower back, pelvic musculature, and abdomen can impair blood flow to reproductive organs. From a yoga perspective, it's particularly important to keep the lumbar spine strong and flexible. Other important targets for our fertility asana are the hip flexors (hip abductors and adductors and psoas), gluteal muscles, the piriformis, and the quadratus lumborum. Stretching these muscles releases the rigid fascia resulting from poor posture, overuse, and injury and improves energy balance and circulation in the pelvic area.

Energy Anatomy

The other benefit of using yoga to help promote fertility is that the practice of hatha yoga provides us with yet another tool for improving fertility. Chakras, which can be visualized as whirling energy centers in the body, are believed by many holistic healers to play a key role in reproductive health. The knowledge of chakras originated from ancient Hindu mystics more than 2,500 years ago who, through meditation and experience, discovered these important energy centers. Hundreds of chakras exist in the body, but healing science focuses on the seven main chakras located along the axis of the spine. The chakras mark the intersection points of the three main energy currents of the body: the *ida* (feminine), the *pingala* (masculine) and the *susumna* (main). Chakras function as wheels, drawing in the life-energy (also called prana, ki or Qi) circulating along these main energy channels and distributing it to the glands, organs, blood, and nervous system of the physical body. Interestingly, each of the seven chakras corresponds to an endocrine gland, physiological function, and specific anatomical region of the physical body.

Chakras are also an archetype for human emotional and spiritual development. Each chakra corresponds to a particular evolutionary life lesson. The chakras are aligned vertically on the spine, ascending from the sacrum (root chakra) to the top of the head (crown chakra). In addition to physical illness, pathology in the chakra system can be caused by less-than-skillful handling of these life-lessons or getting bogged down at one stage or another of spiritual/emotional development, thus preventing the chakra from distributing energy to the physical structures under its control. Table 1.1 (see p. 34) shows the chakra system, its endocrine relationship and corresponding life lesson. Yoga asana, mantra (chanting of sacred syllables) and meditation can be used to balance chakra energy.

The lower three chakras are most commonly associated with fertility. Together these three are called the *kanda*, or bulb, and are known as the region of fire. While many of the postures in the Pulling Down the Moon (PDtM) Yoga for Fertility practice focus on the stimulation of these areas, it is also important to improve the even and vibrant flow of life energy through all the chakras along the spine, as a block in any of these energy centers can, like a kink in a garden hose, affect the health of others along the line.

It is outer chakra function that we affect when practicing yoga postures. The asanas or postures cause the stretching or compressing of different areas of the body. By choosing poses carefully, we can direct life energy into the specific chakra centers. As a result, the physical function of the areas associated with each chakra improves. When practice is regular and mindful, the stimulation of the chakra through the physical postures can lead to an improvement in inner chakra function, allowing for psychological and emotional traumas and patterns associated with the chakra to come first to our attention, and ultimately to resolution. Note also that the chakras have a related sensory activity. So, when you practice your yoga, try to engage as many of the senses as possible. You can do this by playing meaningful music, brewing aromatherapy, creating mood lighting with candles, and practicing in an inviting and uncluttered space.

Chakra levels

According to the teachings of the yogic medical science of Ayurveda, there are three levels on which the chakras work:
1. *"Outer" chakra function—relates to physical diseases, nerve plexuses, and endocrine function associated with each chakra.*
2. *"Inner" chakra function—relates to psychological and emotional disease.*
3. *"Opening" the chakras—relates to transcending the ordinary physical and mental function of the chakras and merging with the Supreme Self.*
(Frawley, 1999)

TABLE 1.1 CHAKRA/ENDOCRINE/PHYSIOLOGY

CHAKRA	WHERE?	EVOLUTIONARY LESSON	SENSORY ACTION	ENDOCRINE GLAND	ACTION IN THE BODY
First Chakra *Muladhara* "root chakra"	Sacrum	Our sense of safety, security, trust, relationship with family, money, job, home	Smell	Adrenals	Sacrum, legs, bones, feet, rectum, and immune system
Second Chakra *Svadisthana*	Pelvis	Sensations, feeling, food, sex, appetite	Taste	Gonads: Ovaries and Testes	Sex organs, lower back, pelvis, appendix, bladder and hips, large intestine
Third Chakra *Manipura*	Solar Plexus	Personal power, ego, self-efficacy, freedom, intellect	Vision	Pancreas	Stomach, small intestine, liver, gallbladder, spleen, mid-spine
Fourth Chakra *Anahata*	Heart	Love, compassion, gratitude, empathy and forgiveness, relating, giving affection	Touch	Thymus	Heart, circulatory system, respiratory system, breasts, diaphragm, and thorax
Fifth Chakra *Vishuddha*	Throat	Self-expression and concrete manifestation	Hearing	Thyroid	Throat, thyroid, mouth, teeth and gums, esophagus, parathyroid, hypothalamus
Sixth Chakra *Ajna*	Third Eye	Learning to trust intuition, learning about the mind	ESP	Pituitary, hypothalamus	Brain, nervous system, eyes, ears, nose, endocrine system
Seventh Chakra *Sahasrara*	Crown of the Head	Opening to spirituality, exploring divinity	Empathy	Pineal	Muscular system, skeletal system, skin

The Yoga for Fertility Practice

The overall goal of the PDtM Yoga for Fertility practice is five-fold:

1. To learn to deepen and control our breathing for relaxation and stress reduction.
2. To increase flexibility in the hips, groin, lower back, chest, and shoulders.
3. To increase the flow of life-energy (prana) through the chakras.
4. To increase blood flow to the reproductive organs.
5. To stimulate the flow of apana and samana, two energy currents in the body which are important for optimal fertility (see box, opposite).

The practice has four sections:

1. Breath awareness practices
2. Kriya (cleansing) exercises
3. Asana practices
4. Relaxation

Apana and Samana

The prana vayus—apana, samana, prana, udana, and vyana—*are the five energy currents in the body that describe the flow of life energy. While each of these is present and important for physiological and spiritual function, our main emphasis in fertility yoga is to stimulate the healthy flow of apana and samana.*

- Apana vayu *flows downward and outward, and is the energy that supports healthy menstruation and the elimination of toxins. On a psycho-spiritual level, apana governs the expulsion of negative sensory, emotional, and mental experiences, or "toxins of the mind." When apana is weak or misdirected, the result is greed, fear, and depression. When strong, apana strengthens our capacity for detachment and dispassion, and functions as our internal "reality check," constantly returning us to a sense* of grounding and connection with our essential Self.

- Samana vayu *flows from the periphery to the center of the abdomen and encourages digestion and assimilation of food, as well as the absorption of oxygen in the lungs. Psycho-spiritually, samana allows for the "digestion" of information and experiences by the mind. When samana is weak or "deranged," we lose the abilities of mental concentration, balance, and discrimination.*

In most beginner yogis and the general population, apana and samana vayus are feeble and diminished by poor eating, sleeping and exercise patterns. By improving our diet and digestion, and using specific yoga postures, we can strengthen the vayus and improve their associated functions.

If you work through all four sections, your practice will take about 50 minutes. For a shorter practice, the breathing and kriya exercises can be done on their own. Before beginning this or any other yoga program, always check with your physician first to make sure it's appropriate for you.

Each section is described on the following pages. Take time to learn about the different practices, their energetic effects and effects on the physical body. In yoga, we say, "energy follows intention." In other words, the more aware you are of the effects and objectives of different poses or techniques, the more profoundly you will benefit from them.

This yoga program is safe to follow during Assisted Reproductive Technology (ART) cycles with the exception of the 48 hours post-IVF retrieval and 48 hours post-IVF embryo transfer. In addition, be aware that ovarian stimulation can cause pain and distention in the abdomen. It is important *not* to practice yoga if you are experiencing pain as a result of stimulation medication. The restorative postures on pp. 150–1 are a good option for any phase in your ART cycle.

BREATH AWARENESS PRACTICES

In this section we will first learn to feel our breath in our bodies and use the *awareness of the breath* to help us find where we may be storing our stress, tensions, toxins, and emotions. This new, conscious breathing is fertility-friendly breathing and can be used as a preparation for asana practice as well as during other stressful life situations. We will also learn the *ujayii breath*, or victorious breath. Ujayii is an active, stimulating breathing technique that builds a gentle heat in the body called tapas. We will use ujayii during the asana portion of practice. Since breathing nourishes and stimulates the chakras, you may want to return to the chakra chart and refresh your understanding of these energy centers and their significance and functions.

Exercise 1: Finding your breath

Lie down on your back and bend your knees so that the soles of the feet are on the floor, hip-width apart. Allow the knees to rest in on each other. Place your hands on the base of your belly. Begin to breathe through your nose.

With your next inhale, draw the breath deep into your low belly. Feel your hands rise with the breath, and then exhale completely. Repeat several times, softening the muscles of the belly and back to allow the lower pelvis to fill completely with breath and prana. This may take some practice and you may discover that this area feels tight or blocked. Use your inhales to create space, and use your exhales to release stress, tension, toxins and emotions that might be stored in this area. As you become more adept, you can begin to breathe even deeper, ultimately as if you are touching the breath to the soles of your feet. Be patient, continuing to breathe down to the pelvic floor, legs, and feet. Notice any sensation without judging. *Notice also how breathing down deep into your low belly makes you feel. Breathing in this way helps to ground us emotionally. We nourish the first and second chakras when breathing in this way.*

Complete 12 repetitions of these low belly breaths.

Now gently shift your hands to the middle ribs. Breathe into this area, the solar plexus, feeling the ribcage as it expands from side to side and from forward to back. Again, use your inhales to create space, and use exhales to release tension, toxins, and emotions. *Notice how breathing into the solar plexus helps to create space around emotions that "tighten the gut." Breathing into the solar plexus helps to nourish the third chakra, often the receptacle of anger and frustration.*

Complete 12 repetitions of these mid-rib breaths.

Now shift your hands up to rest just below your collarbone. Breathe up into your upper chest. Feel the breath move into your heart center and notice any physical sensations of tightness or tension, either in front or in the back, between the shoulder blades. As the breath becomes fuller in the upper chest, you can begin to move the breath upward into the throat, to the brow, to the crown of your head. *Notice how breathing into the heart center helps to make space around anxiety or sadness that might be lodged in the heart center. As the breath moves upward into the throat and head, feel it clearing obsessive thoughts and emotions and creating clarity.*

Complete 12 repetitions of these upper-chest breaths.

Now, begin to take slow, full breaths that sequentially fill the lower belly, middle ribs, and upper chest, pausing as you fill each zone. Exhale in the same way, emptying the lower belly then the middle ribs, then the upper chest, again pausing as you empty each zone.

Complete 12 repetitions of these full, three-part breaths.

You can add a pelvic tilt here to create a soothing, rocking sensation in the abdominal area. As you inhale, allow the pelvis to tilt forward until there is the slightest arch in your lower back—enough to slip a hand beneath the small of the back. As you exhale, ground the low back and allow the pelvis to tip slightly back, tail bone lifting just off the floor.

Exercise 2: Ujayii breath

Sit in a comfortable position. Hold your hand in front of your mouth as if it is a mirror. Take a deep breath through your nose in and then exhale through your mouth on to your hand, making a "Haa" sound, as if fogging up the mirror. Try this a few times.

Now try the same breath, but this time close the mouth on your exhale, still making the "Haa" sound. Now it becomes a low, soft hiss in the back of your throat. Try to breathe in through your nose in the same way, creating that gentle hissing sound in the back of the throat. Practice until you can inhale and exhale smoothly, making the hissing sound on both the in and out breaths.

This ujayii breath serves several key purposes in our practice. First, as mentioned earlier, it creates a subtle heat, called tapas, that purifies the energy channels of our body. Second, the ujayii vibration is localized in the throat near the soft palate. Just behind this area is the master fertility gland, the hypothalamus. It is believed that the subtle vibration of the ujayii breath stimulates and promotes blood flow to this important endocrine gland. Finally, the ujayii breath is audible and serves as a place for us to tether our wandering attention while we do our yoga. At all times during practice you should be listening to the sound of the breath. It is this focus on the breath that turns yoga from a simple stretching routine into a meditative practice.

Poses and their Effects: The Specific Yoga Asanas

Since one of our most important tenets is that energy follows intention, let's take time before practice to discuss the different elements of practice and understand why they are important for our health and fertility. In general, different kinds of yoga postures have different physiological and energetic effects:

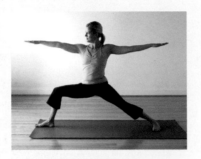

Standing poses *help to stretch and strengthen the lower body and spine. These poses create a sense of balance and rooted-ness. Through these poses, we "find our feet" and "get out of our heads." Standing postures increase apana and can nourish and strengthen the menstrual cycle.*

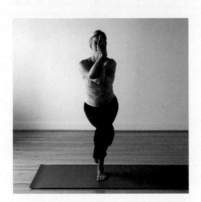

Balance poses *help to improve our connection with our feet and our core. They often reveal imbalances in our bodily structure. On an energetic level, balance poses challenge us to clear our mind and remain calm on shaky ground.*

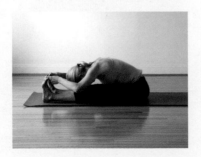

Forward folds *help to release tight hamstrings and lower backs and serve to increase blood flow into the pelvis. Energetically, forward folds are calming in effect. These poses decrease sympathetic tone in the body and promote parasympathetic activities like digestion and elimination.*

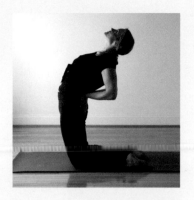

Backbends strengthen and stretch the musculature in the back body, neck, and shoulders. Backbends are energetically stimulating and good mood elevators.

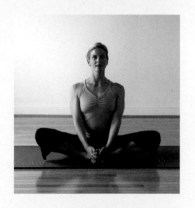

Hip openers focus on the tight muscles and fascia in and around the hip joints and help to reduce chronic tension in the low back. In addition, stretching in the hips allows for greater blood flow into the pelvic organs as well as improved nerve transmission to the nerve plexuses of the lower sacrum. From a yogic anatomy standpoint, the hips are where we store a great deal of emotion and disappointment.

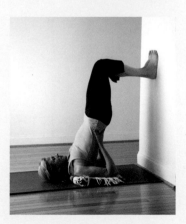

Inversions are poses that place the head below the heart and promote profound changes in circulation and mental perspective. They include headstand, shoulder stand (shown), and viparita karani (legs up the wall), among others. Inversions (excluding viparita karani) should not be practiced during menses.

KRIYA (CLEANSING) EXERCISES

Kriya are cleansing exercises that help to dislodge toxicity and open important energy channels. These particular kriya are fertility-specific and stimulate the musculature and fascia of the low back, hips, and the feet, opening the apana energy channel. Hips and feet are linked to the downward flow of energy that helps to ground us and make us feel emotionally secure. These exercises can be done daily.

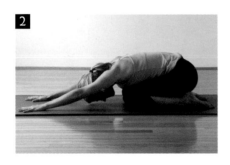

• *Chakra Vrksasana*

Chakra Vrksasana is a wonderful warm-up for the low back, hips, and breath. This three-part kriya exercise is done in two phases:

1. Begin in Table Pose, on your hands and knees
2. Take a deep inhale and then exhale, round your back like an angry cat and sit your seat back on to your heels (Child Pose).
3. With your next inhale, return to Table Pose.

Repeat 4 times, using your breath to set the pace of the movement.

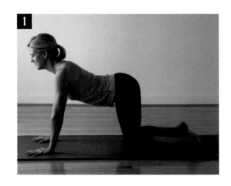

Try to take your time moving between Table Pose and Child Pose, feeling the spine as it rounds and the muscles of the back becoming warm. Feel how the breath and the movement become synchronized.

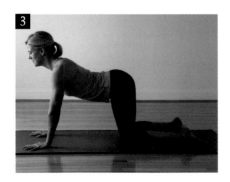

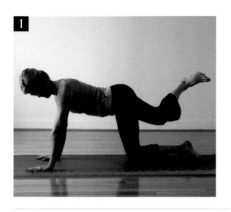

- **Hip Circles**
1. From Table Pose, lift the right leg with knee bent 90 degrees and make full circles in the hip joint. Do this with the intention of "clearing out cobwebs" in the hip sockets. Rest in Child Pose.
2. Bring your awareness to the sole of the right foot. Perhaps it is more "alive" than before.
3. Now move the left side. Bring your awareness to the sole of the left foot. Perhaps it is more "alive" than before.

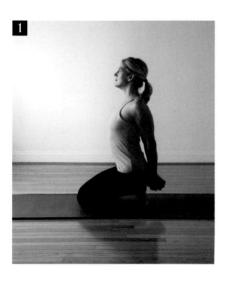

- **Stretching the Sole**
1. Stand on your knees, curl toes under and sit your seat back gently on to the heels. If the soles of your feet or your toes are very tight, this may be quite uncomfortable. Never force, go gently. The soles of the feet are important conduits for apana energy, the energy that supports fertility.
2. Next, move back into table and gently tap the tops of the feet on the floor, massaging and encouraging blood and energy flow into tight toes and ankles.

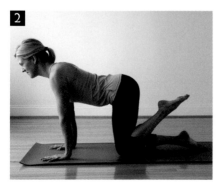

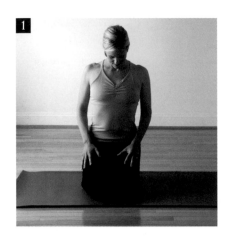

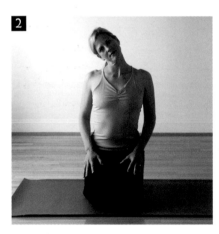

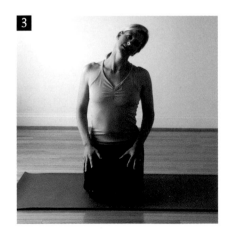

• *Neck Rolls*

1. Gently drop your head, chin to chest.
2. Now make a soft arc to the right, drawing the right ear towards the right shoulder. Linger in any part of the range of motion that feels tight or tense.
3. Gently roll to the other side.

Repeat.

ASANA PRACTICES

Once you have completed 5–10 minutes of Breath Awareness practice and 5 minutes of Kriya (Cleansing) Exercises, it is time to "build" your yoga asana practice, which should consist of:

• PDtM Moon Salutes (2–4 rounds)
• One of the therapeutic sessions—Hip/Heart Opening or Digestion/Hormonal Balance

After this you will enter the last section of Yoga for Fertility practice, the relaxation phase. This is also known as the Final Resting Pose or Svasana (5–10 minutes).

Moon Salutes

The PDtM practice begins with 2–4 rounds PDtM's Moon Salutes (see pages 44 and 45). This series of postures, which links breath and movement, effects a gentle warming in the body as well as helps to transition the mind into a more meditative state. The linking of breath and movement is called *vinyasa* and as you become more adept with your yoga practice you may actually feel your breath beginning to lead your body from pose to pose. As opposed to the more commonly known and more vigorous Surya Namaskar (Sun Salutation), this moon salute uses squats, folds, and lunges to stimulate blood flow into the pelvis and legs, to calm the mind and to strengthen apana vayu.

Do 2–4 rounds of Moon Salutes (one round = once through on each side). Focus on the ujayii breath and the flow of postures. From your final Tadasana (Mountain) Pose go directly into the therapeutic session of your choice.

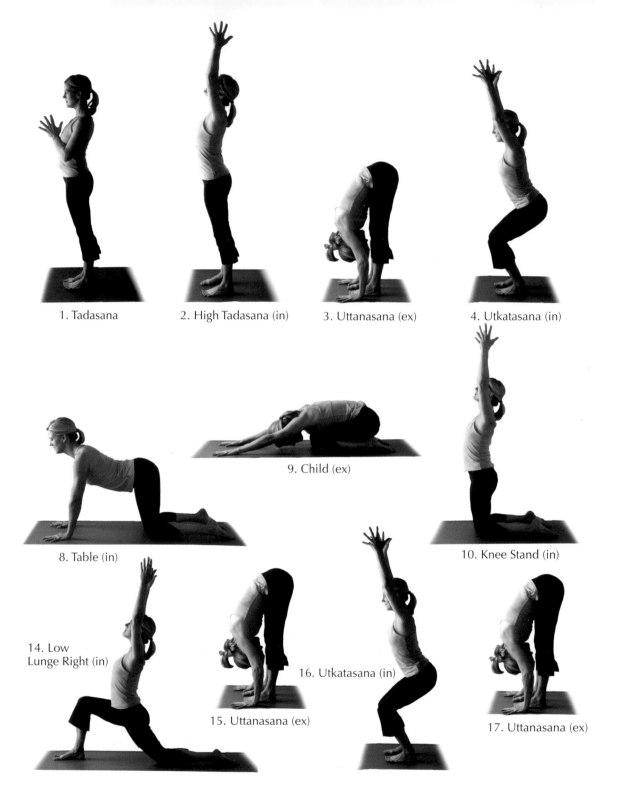

1. Tadasana

2. High Tadasana (in)

3. Uttanasana (ex)

4. Utkatasana (in)

8. Table (in)

9. Child (ex)

10. Knee Stand (in)

14. Low Lunge Right (in)

15. Uttanasana (ex)

16. Utkatasana (in)

17. Uttanasana (ex)

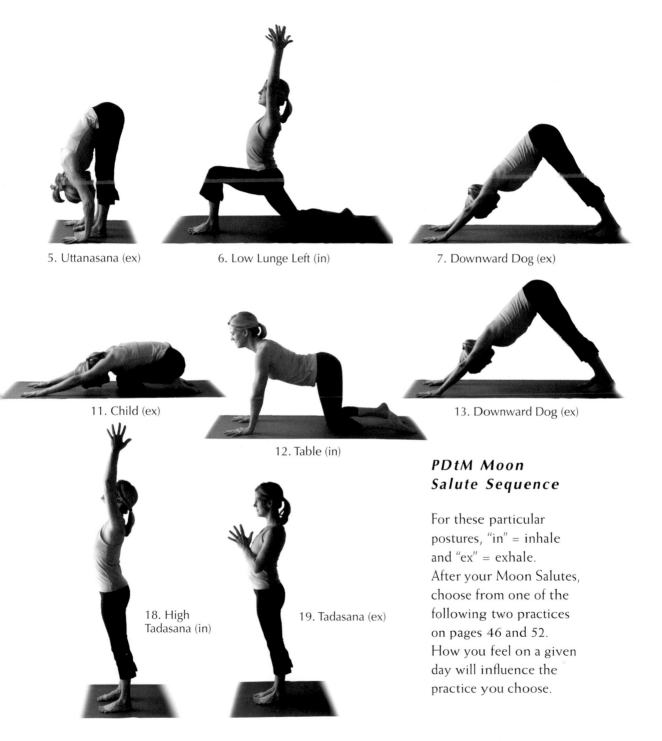

5. Uttanasana (ex)

6. Low Lunge Left (in)

7. Downward Dog (ex)

11. Child (ex)

12. Table (in)

13. Downward Dog (ex)

18. High Tadasana (in)

19. Tadasana (ex)

PDtM Moon Salute Sequence

For these particular postures, "in" = inhale and "ex" = exhale. After your Moon Salutes, choose from one of the following two practices on pages 46 and 52. How you feel on a given day will influence the practice you choose.

Asana Practice 1: Hips and Heart Opening
Apana/Prana Practice

The first practice to open hips and heart includes standing postures to ground the energy in the legs and feet and improve the flow of apana energy in the body. This practice also uses shoulder stretches and supported backbends to release anxiety.

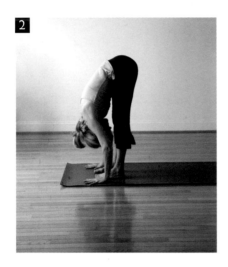

• *Uttanasana/Utkatasana Vinyasa*

1. Stand with your feet hip-distance apart at the top of your mat, hands on hips.
2. Inhale, then with your exhale, hinge forward into Forward Fold. Knees will be bent or straight, depending on your hamstring flexibility.
3. With your next inhale, bend your knees and sit your seat into Chair Pose. Hold for 3 breaths.

Repeat 2 more times.

This vinyasa helps to build a gentle heat (tapas) in the body as well as strengthen the apana vayu. The forward fold releases tension in the lower back and stimulates the second chakra, or fertility chakra.

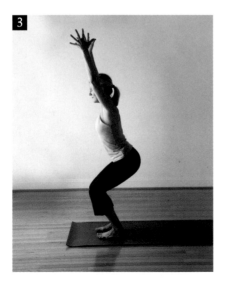

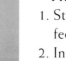

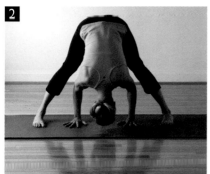

• Prasarita Padottanasana with Squats

1. Stand with your feet spread wide on your mat, feet parallel.
2. Inhale, then fold forward into Prasarita Padottanasana. Hold here and breathe for several breaths.
3. Now walk your hands forward about 2 feet and gently press your weight back in space.
4. With an inhale, take a squat in Prasarita Padottanasana.

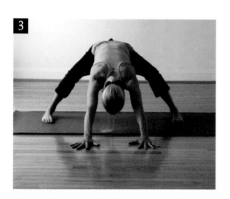

The squat may be a small movement, depending on hip flexibility, and it may feel like you're just plain stuck. Don't judge, just observe the sensation as it arises.

Focus on the breath as you repeat sequence 2–3 times.

This vinyasa stretches hamstrings, groin muscles, and deep hip flexors. Notice how your hips "hum" when you're finished with this one.

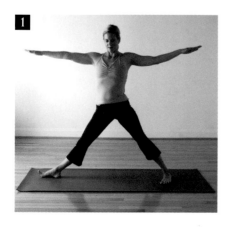

• Dynamic Virabhadrasana II

1. From the previous pose, turn your right toes out 90 degrees, and angle your left toes towards the right. Check your alignment. If you drew a line from the right heel to the left foot it would bisect the left arch. Extend arms out in opposite directions, shoulder height.

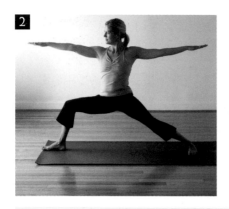

2. Take an inhale, and with your next exhale, bend your right knee 90 degrees.

Repeat 4 times on the right side, inhaling the right leg straight, exhaling right knee bent. Now do the other side.

Virabhadrasana II translates as Warrior Pose. This is a fabulous fertility pose. In addition to stimulating apana, it also helps to strengthen and stretch the muscles of our legs. This pose also challenges us to find the subtle balance between hard work and effortlessness.

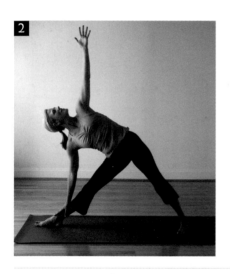

• Trikonasana

1. From Virabhadrasana II, straighten your right leg and narrow your stance a bit. Again, turn your right toes out 90 degrees, and angle your left toes towards the right.
2. Take an inhale and with your exhale, place the right hand down on your shin, extending the left hand skyward. Take 5–10 breaths.

Repeat on the other side.

Trikonasana stretches hips, groin, and low back. In addition, the pose is a wonderful heart opener and reduces chronic tension in the upper back.

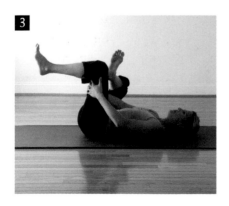

• Number Four/Supta Hasta Padangusthasana

This pose is called Number Four Pose because the leg configuration resembles the number "4." To do the pose:

1. Lay on your back with your knees bent, feet on the floor, hip-distance apart.
2. Cross your right ankle on to your left knee.
3. Now lift your left foot (bottom leg) off the floor and draw the left thigh towards the body. You can interlace your fingers behind the left thigh to help

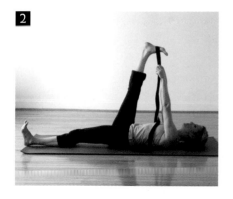

encourage the stretch. You should *not* feel this in the knee of the crossed leg. If you do, place the bottom foot back on the ground and enjoy the stretch here. Hold for 10–20 deep breaths.

Now move into Supta Hasta Padangusthasana:
1. Stretch your left leg along the floor and put your yoga strap around the sole of the right foot. Extend the foot to the ceiling.
2. Gently stretch the leg as straight as possible without straining, and flex the right foot.
3. Hold 5–10 breaths.
4. Now take both ends of the strap into the right hand and lower the right leg out to the side until you feel a good stretch in the right inner thigh. Keep left hip/buttocks grounded.
5. Hold for 5–10 breaths.
6. Bring leg back up and hug it into your chest.

Repeat series beginning with the Number Four Pose on the left side.

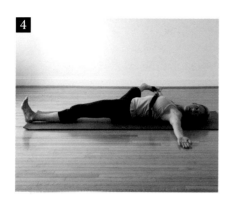

• *Baddha Konasana*

1. Sit up straight with the soles of your feet touching, knees apart (you can sit on a folded blanket if it is difficult to sit on the floor with a straight spine).
2. Take hold of the feet with your hands. Inhale, sit up straight and tall, and exhale, folding forward. Keep your spine as straight as possible as you hinge from the hips. Take 5–10 breaths here.

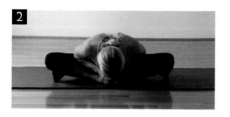

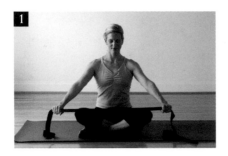

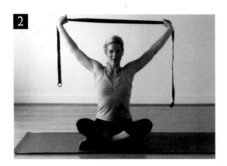

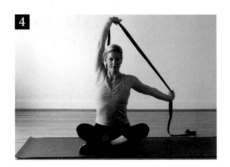

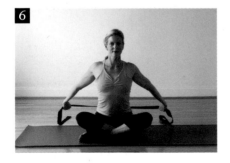

• *Shoulder Series with Strap*

1. Sit in a comfortable seated position and take your yoga strap in both hands, hands about shoulders' width apart.
2. With an inhale, stretch the strap up over your head. Take 5–10 breaths as you stretch your arms gently up and back.
3. Drop the right arm down and bring the left arm up, taking 5–10 breaths. Return arms over head.
4. Drop the left arm down and bring the right arm up, taking 5–10 breaths. Return arms over head.
5. Lower arms to the front.

Now try the "Up-and-Over" Shoulder Stretch:
6. With the same shoulder-width grip on the strap, inhale the arms up and overhead and then exhale the strap down behind your back.
7. Inhale and take the strap overhead, returning to the starting point.

The goal of the up-and-over is to keep the arms straight during the entire range of movement. If you cannot take the strap up and over with straight arms, take a wider grip on the strap. Go slow, take your time at the "sticky" parts and enjoy the sensation as you open tight chest muscles and rediscover lost shoulder mobility.

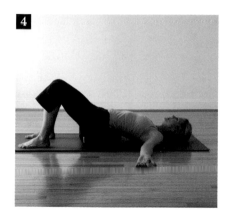

• **Supported Setu Bandhasana**
1. Lie on your back with your knees bent, feet flat on the floor, hip-distance apart.
2. Lift your hips and slide a bolster or 2 rolled blankets under the small of your back and lower hips down. The bolster should support the lower back and there should be no discomfort in the sacral area.
3. Take arms out to the sides, palms facing up.
4. Breathe and fully surrender to gravity and allow the bolster to support and nurture your lower back. Deeply release in the pelvis and buttocks. Hold here up to 5 minutes.

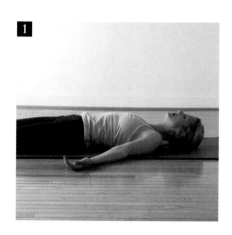

RELAXATION, OR SVASANA

Svasana is the most important pose of our yoga practice. In Svasana all the physical, energetic, and emotional work of practice is processed and our bodies have time to rest and restore. It is a time of profound "not-doing" as well as an opportunity to surrender to something greater than ourselves (see Prayer p. 216).
1. Lie on your back, legs and arms straight, palms facing up. If the lower back feels uncomfortable in this position, place a bolster under your knees.
2. Starting at your feet, scan your body for any residual tension. If you find any places that are restless or tense, breathe into them and allow them to relax with your exhale.
3. Let go of the effort of being in the physical body. Allow your body to become very heavy.
4. Let go of the effort of breathing. Release the ujayii breath and let the breath breathe you.
5. Let go of effort of thought. Choose not to attach to the thoughts that wander through your head.
6. Now let everything go—body, mind and spirit—surrendering to the present moment.

Asana Practice 2: Hormonal Regulation/Digestion Improvement Samana Practice

The goal of this practice is to balance the endocrine system, improve digestion and the assimilation of nutrients (samana vayu) as well as speed up the elimination of toxins. The gentle twists in this practice are safe for the fertility process and will help to release tension in the abdomen, improve blood flow to the abdominal region and stimulate digestion.

Shoulder Stand and Supported Fish stimulate the thyroid gland by first compressing (Shoulder Stand), then stretching (Supported Fish) the throat area. The thyroid gland is essential for good hormonal function and strong metabolism. Practicing Shoulder Stand in this way is also quite calming, and it stimulates our body's "rest and digest" hormone system. This is also known as the autonomic hormone system.

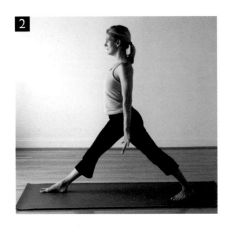

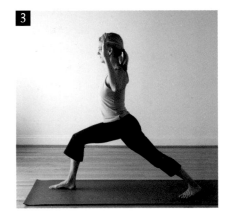

• Dynamic Virabhadrasana I

Also known as Warrior I, this standing pose creates strength and flexibility in the hips, shoulders, and upper back. As you practice the dynamic vinyasa, you may feel heat building in your body.

1. Stand, feet together, at the front of your mat. Take a big step backward with your left foot, about 3½ feet.
2. Keep your right toes facing forward, angle left toes slightly left, about 45 degrees. Hands hang down at your sides. Try to square your hips forward.
3. With an inhale, bend the right knee as close to 90 degrees as possible. At the same time, raise your arms to a "double cactus" position, elbows bent and palms facing forward.
4. Exhale and straighten the right leg, lowering arms. Repeat this 5 times and on the last repetition, hold bent leg position and take 10 breaths.

Repeat on the left.

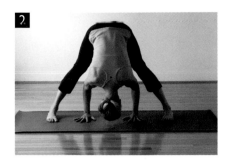

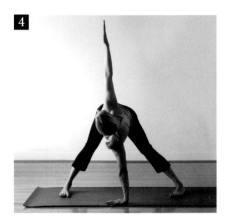

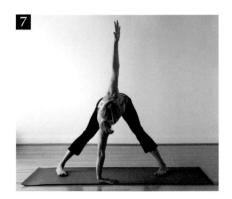

• *Prasarita Padottanasana with Twist*

Also known as Wide Leg Forward Bend, this pose stretches the groin and hamstrings. When we add the twist element, we make the spine more supple as well as stimulate the abdominal organs.

1. Stand with feet spread wide on your mat, feet parallel.
2. Inhale, then fold forward into Wide Leg Forward Bend. Hold here and take several breaths.
3. Place your left hand on the floor under your nose, with your fingers facing to the right. You can place your hand on a block if you have difficulty keeping your knees straight.
4. With an inhale, stretch your right hand up to the sky, gently twisting in the upper back. As you breathe here, try and stack the right shoulder directly above the left.
5. Press down into both feet, reach back through your tailbone and forward through the crown of your head. Find the current of energy that runs from the left hand up through the right fingertips.
6. Take 5–10 breaths. Release to center with an exhale. Rest a moment and enjoy the sensation.
7. Now place the right hand on the floor (or on a block) under your nose and reach skyward with the left. Again, locate all the currents of energy flowing here, downward through the soles of the feet, along the spine from the tailbone to head and through the heart from palm to palm.
8. Take 5–10 breaths here and then release again to center.

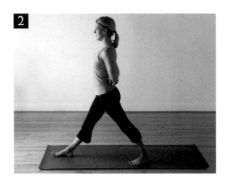

• *Parsvottanasana*

You may find you struggle with balance in this pose, which is also called Pyramid Pose. This standing asana stretches hips, hamstrings, and low back. In addition, the forward fold nourishes and stimulates the lower abdomen and belly.

1. Stand at the front of your mat, feet together. Take a step backward with your left foot, about 2½ feet.
2. Keep your right toes facing forward, turn the left toes out about 45 degrees to the left. Square hips forward.
3. Reach your arms out to the sides with an inhale and with your exhale, grab opposite elbows behind your back.
4. Inhale and then exhale, allowing your torso to fold forward into Parsvottanasana. Keep squaring your hips forward. Breathe here for 5–10 breaths.
5. With an inhale, come up with a straight spine.

Repeat other side.

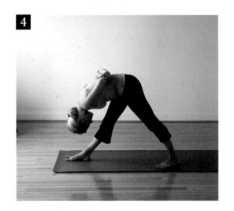

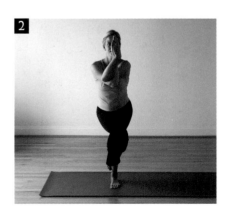

• *Garudasana (Eagle Pose)*

Eagle pushes blood from the extremities into the abdomen, nourishing organs of digestion and reproduction. It detoxifies by compressing lymph nodes in the armpits and groin.

1. From standing, bend your left knee slightly and shift weight into the left leg and lift the right leg up, wrapping the right thigh around the left, hooking the right foot behind the left ankle.
2. Now bend your elbows and lift them to shoulder level. Cross the left elbow over the right and hook the right wrist and palm over the left. Hold for 10 breaths.

Repeat other side

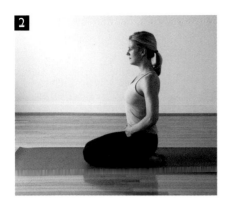

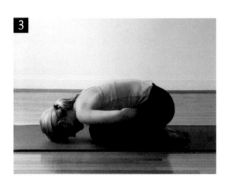

• *Vadhrasana with Abdominal Massage*

Omit this pose if you are taking ovarian stimulation drugs, are post-ovulation, post-retrieval, or if there is any chance that you may be pregnant.

1. Come into a kneeling position, tops of the feet on the floor beneath your seat. If you experience discomfort in your knees or the tops of the feet you may place a blanket under your seat.

2. Make fists with your hands and place them in the crease between your thigh and torso.

3. Inhale and then exhale your torso forward over your fists.

4. Gently move the fists around in circles, kneading the lower abdomen.

5. Inhale, come back up, and move the fists higher so the knuckles meet in front of the navel.

6. Inhale and with an exhale fold forward again, this time using the compressed fists to gently massage the middle of the belly.

7. Inhale, come back up, and shift the fists higher on the belly so that they rest on the fleshy part of the belly just below the ribcage.

8. With your next exhale, fold forward again, massaging the upper abdomen just below the diaphragm muscle.

9. Inhale back to seated and notice the sensation of energy in the belly.

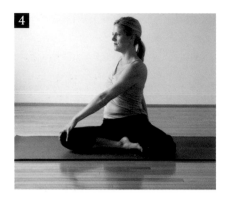

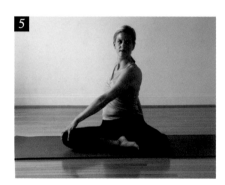

• *Bharadvajasana*

This pose is a wonderful twist for all individuals, and is safe for any phase of the fertility cycle. It is also one of the only safe twists during pregnancy. Rishi means "divinely inspired sage" in Sanskrit and this twist helps us become aware of our innate wisdom and compassion.

1. Begin seated with legs outstretched in front of you. Sit on a blanket if it's difficult to keep a straight spine.

2. Bring the heel of your right foot into the groin, with the sole of the foot against the inner left thigh, and fold the left leg alongside the body. The top of the left foot should be tucked along the left hip, the sole of the left foot facing the ceiling.

3. With the heel of the right foot pressing firmly against the pelvic floor and both sitting bones fully grounded, sit tall. Move your attention down toward the floor through the perinueum and sitting bones and then lift your ribcage away from your hip bones, gently pulling belly button to spine. The front knee can gently lift away from the floor in order to firmly ground the sitting bones.

4. Reach your right hand behind you to the floor. Inhale the left arm up by the ear and with an exhale take the left hand to the right knee.

5. Inhale again, making the spine long and tall and then exhale, twisting the torso and shoulders to the right and looking gently over the left shoulder. Do not torque or strain the neck here.

6. Take 10–20 breaths here, inhales making the spine long, exhales deepening the twist.

7. Gently release the pose and stretch the legs forward, bouncing them gently.

Repeat other side.

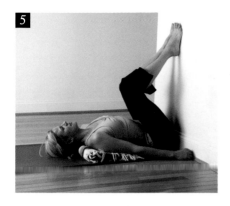

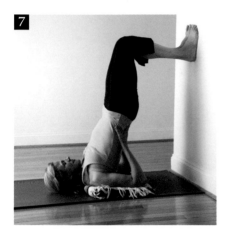

• *Salamba Sarvangasana (Supported Shoulder Stand)*

We do not recommend practicing inversions during your menstrual period. If you are menstruating, we suggest you do Viparita Karani (p.150) instead.

1. Lie on the floor with your legs up the wall, sitting bones as close to the wall as possible.
2. Take note of where your shoulders are on your mat and then come back to a seated position.
3. Place your folded blanket where your shoulders will be.
4. Now, lie down again with legs up the wall, sitting bones as close to the wall as possible. The blanket should support your shoulders and the back of the head should be on the floor. Play a bit until you get the support just right.
5. Slide your feet down until the soles of the feet are flat on the wall.
6. With an inhale, lift the hips, tuck the pelvis in, and press the soles of the feet into the wall. Gently roll the shoulders under and move the shoulder blades towards each other as you lift into Supported Shoulder Stand.
7. Walk the feet up the wall until the shins are parallel to the floor and bring the hands to support the lower back.
8. Breathe here, continuing to ground the shoulders down, scoop the tailbone, and bring the chest closer to the chin.
9. Hold for 20–30 breaths.

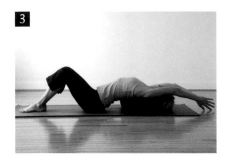

• *Supported Matsyasana (Fish)*

This counter-pose to Supported Shoulder Stand is wonderful for balancing the thyroid as well as opening the heart center to release sadness and anxiety. You will need a bolster or a rolled blanket to do this restorative pose.

1. Sit on your yoga mat with your knees bent, soles of your feet on the floor.
2. Lie back onto a bolster or rolled blanket so that the bolster is supporting your upper back and your head is free to stretch back and rest on the floor. If it feels uncomfortable to lie like this, or if the stretch feels too intense on your neck, place a towel under the head to lessen the bend in the neck.
3. Take your hands in front of the heart in prayer and then stretch them up over your head toward the floor.
4. Take 10–20 breaths.
5. To come out of the pose, bring your hands back to your heart and then release them on the floor. Gently scoot your shoulders off the bolster so your head is now resting on the support, as on a pillow.
6. Roll to your right side and rest here for a few breaths before returning to seated.

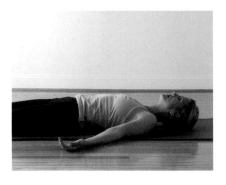

RELAXATION, OR SVASANA

Svasana is the final, and most important, pose of our yoga practice. In Svasana all the physical, energetic and emotional work of practice is processed and our bodies have time to rest and restore. See page 51 for more details.

Physical Activity Guidelines for Assisted Reproductive Technology (ART) Patients

Physical activity may relieve stress, elevate mood and help to moderate many of the side effects of fertility medications (bloating, headache, mood swings, etc.). Patients can maintain moderate levels of physical activity prior to and during ART cycles, with a few simple modifications.

Pre-stimulation:
- *Moderate physical activity is appropriate when preparing for ART.*
- *Moderate exercise is considered to be 3–4 exercise sessions per week for 30–45 minutes per session.*
- *Recommended exercises: low-impact activities such as walking, swimming, yoga, biking, and strength training.*
- *There is some clinical evidence that intense aerobic exercise (running, spinning) may disrupt reproductive hormone regulation.*

During stimulation:
- *Continue with mild physical activity (shorter, less intense sessions) as long as you are not experiencing discomfort or pain in the pelvic area.*
- *If you are experiencing pelvic discomfort, stop! Lower the intensity of your workouts and avoid abdominal crunches and twists. If discomfort is severe or persists, always consult your physician.*

Post-retrieval:
- *Patients differ enormously in their experience of egg retrieval. Some experience a significant amount of discomfort and swelling, while others experience little or no effects at all.*
- *48 hours of rest (see note below) is advised immediately post-retrieval to allow for any discomfort to subside.*
- *Wait until any swelling, discomfort, or inflammation dissipates before resuming even mild physical activity.*

Post-transfer:
- *48 hours of rest (see note) is usually advised immediately post-transfer.*
- *After 48 hours, the resumption of gentle physical activity is permissible in the absence of pain, inflammation, or other side effects of treatment.*
- *Gentle, low-impact activity (walking, swimming, yoga) during the "two-week wait" period is appropriate.*
- *Physical activity will not impede embryo implantation or make it "fall out."*
- *If any activity causes pain or discomfort, stop!*
- *Avoid becoming short of breath, dehydrated, or over-heated. Your pulse rate should be no more than 60% of the "target" pulse (usually 120 beats per minute).*
- *Avoid hot baths or Jacuzzis.*

Note: Rest is defined as "take it easy." Stay on the couch, watch movies, read, sit in the yard. If your job allows you time to sit and relax, you can return—if your job requires any heavy activity, you may request a note for "light duty."

Beyond Yoga: Fertility-Friendly Exercise

Has it ever run through your mind that perhaps you need to give up all exercise in order to get pregnant? The answer to this question is a resounding "no!" Exercise has been shown to relieve depression, control stress, and help women maintain a healthy body weight—all of which are important for fertility. What you do need to consider, however, is how to exercise in a way that is "fertility friendly," and that may mean lowering the intensity of your exercise, incorporating exercise modalities that focus on anabolic (building) rather than catabolic (burning) processes, and ensuring that you get adequate nutrition, sleep, and rest/recovery time to balance your exercise regimen.

Intensity

When we talk about exercise intensity we are talking about how hard your body works during a particular exercise activity. There are two easy ways to think about exercise intensity—the first is in terms of energy balance and the second is in terms of impact.

Intensity of an exercise determines its energy requirement, or how many calories we burn while exercising. High intensity exercise can be detrimental to fertility. The first way in which exercise can negatively impact fertility is by creating a negative energy balance in women who do not need to lose weight. Energy balance is a simple equation that

Guidelines for Fertility-Friendly Workouts

- *Avoid high-impact/high-intensity activities like running, spin biking, high-impact aerobics, jumping rope, and kick boxing.*
- *While engaging in cardiovascular exercise, keep heart rate at < 60 percent maximum.*

220 – AGE = Estimated Maximum Heart Rate
(Estimated Maximum Heart Rate) x 0.60 = Upper Limit for Fertility-Friendly Exercise

- *Exercise at a lower intensity for a longer duration.*
- *Resistance training (working with weights) is low-impact and does not produce high levels of endorphins. Strength training can also help to create muscle tone and shape, as well as support bone health.*
- *Try to slow down and enjoy your exercise sessions.*
- *Use exercise as a time to unwind—get outside and walk or take a leisurely bike ride.*
- *Explore other non-traditional exercise methods including T'ai Chi, NIA and low-impact aerobic classes like salsa aerobics and ballet fitness.*

nutritionists and exercise physiologists use to conceptualize the factors at work in weight loss and weight gain. The energy balance equation is:

When Energy In = Energy Out, body weight is stable
When Energy In > Energy Out, there is weight gain
When Energy In < Energy Out, there is weight loss

The catch is that negative energy balance in females is associated with decreases in circulating metabolic hormones (like thyroid hormone) that regulate overall metabolic rate, and with increases in baseline levels of stress hormones such as cortisol. Often, shifts in energy balance can occur without weight loss. In such cases, hormonal shifts like the ones described above can be the only indication that a woman is in negative balance. Other signs that a woman may be in negative energy balance are anovulatory cycles or the absence of menstrual periods (amenorrhea).

Now, for women who are overweight, this is not such an area of concern. However, for women who are close to their ideal body weight, a strenuous exercise program might push them into a "sub-fertile" condition. New research recently published in the journal *Obstetrics and Gynecology* reports that women who exercised 4 or more hours per week for 1 to 9 years were 40 percent less likely to have a live birth than women who did not report exercise. These women who exercised heavily were also three times more likely to experience IVF cycle cancellation and twice as likely to have an implantation failure or pregnancy loss.

This research reinforces previous data showing that strenuous exercise can disrupt reproductive hormone regulation. (*Morris, 2006*)

Impact

Exercise is either low- or high-impact. High-impact activity is exercise in which both feet leave the ground. Examples of high-impact exercise are running, aerobic dance that involves jumping, and jumping rope. In general, high-impact exercise can be detrimental to fertility in one of two ways. The first is through the production of endorphins.

Endorphins are the "natural pain killers" produced by the body in response to strenuous exercise. While these chemicals serve to mask pain signals and allow us to enjoy long-duration, strenuous exercise, they can also disrupt reproductive hormone regulation. From the PDtM perspective, the answer is not giving up exercise. Rather, we encourage our patients to examine their current exercise regimen to make sure they are using exercise in a way that supports fertility. The guidelines on the adjacent page are useful for choosing healthy, fertility-friendly workouts. This is not the time to set lofty fitness goals or train for a marathon. Remember, the objective of holistic fertility is to fill yourself with life energy.

Exercise Addiction

Exercise should leave you feeling relaxed and energized—not exhausted. Nor should it cause anxiety. If slowing down your exercise regimen causes you emotional distress, you may want to examine your relationship to physical exercise. If you recognize signs of compulsion or addiction, it may be helpful to discuss this with a mental health professional.

WEEK 1 ACTIVITY 1: AMA CLEANSE

A regular yoga practice will begin to help you dispel both physical and mental toxins. Try this safe, simple 7-day cleanse technique from the yogic medical science of Ayurveda to speed the detoxification of your body systems. *Ama* is a sticky byproduct of poor digestion and toxic living. Ama can cause weakness and inefficiency in our metabolic processes and when left unchecked can begin to cause full-on disease. A combination of yoga asana, a healthy diet (see Week 3), and this 7-day cleanse can help to remove ama from the system.

Sip very hot lemon water frequently throughout the day to dissolve ama:

• Water should be very hot (need to blow on it to drink).

• Squeeze a bit of fresh lemon juice into the water.

• Sip about every 30 minutes (frequency is more important than quantity).

• Drinking 3–4 times a day is not enough—use a large thermos and drink every 30 minutes throughout the day.

Continue this practice for 7 days. This cleanse can be repeated monthly as needed.

Oriental Medicine and the Philosophy of Fertility

SO NOW that you've begun your yoga practice, the journey towards physical, mental, and emotional balance has begun. Even with just one week of yoga, you may be feeling more grounded, calmer, and better able to make positive changes to your lifestyle. This week we're going to look a bit closer at the theory and practice of Oriental Medicine (OM) and consider how this ancient science can improve your fertility. In addition to examining the rationale behind our recommendation of including OM in our Integrative Care for Fertility (ICF) approach, this section will explore the concepts that govern OM and discuss how to integrate these concepts into the Fully Fertile program.

If you're new to the fertility process, some of this information may be new to you. If you've been around the baby-technology block a few times you may have heard or even tried acupuncture for fertility. Either way, we encourage you to read on because this chapter lays the groundwork for other suggestions we'll make later in the book about OM concepts regarding diet, Chinese sexology and Qi Gong and even fertility feng shui. In addition, in this chapter we'll delve deeper into the concept of balance, and how ancient techniques can help us cultivate this elusive quality in our daily lives.

Research Evidence for Oriental Medicine

In April of 2002, a study was published in the medical journal *Fertility and Sterility*, which showed that adding acupuncture to a standard IVF protocol increased pregnancy rates. This study brought acupuncture and OM into the consciousness of the fertility community. The funny thing is that OM practitioners had been treating infertility for years, in fact thousands of years. But the new flurry of interest and investigation brought these ancient healing practices into the limelight.

What the Research Shows

In this study, which is known as the "German Study," researchers examined 160 women who were divided into two groups. Both groups underwent IVF protocol with a day-three embryo transfer. One group also received two acupuncture treatments: one before and one after embryo transfer. The success rate of implantation in those who received acupuncture was 42.5 percent, compared to 26.3 percent for the control group. The result was an increase of 16.2 percent. See Appendix D for more research on acupuncture and fertility.

Obviously, these were exciting results! Since the appearance of this study, there has been much speculation and investigation into how acupuncture can increase fertility. Not long after, pop culture also caught on and Charlotte from Sex in the City was seen hurrying to an acupuncture appointment to help her conceive. The accompanying attention has meant that both the general public and the reproductive medicine community have become acquainted with the potential of these ancient healing techniques, which is great.

Despite these encouraging results, there are still critics. Clinical studies using OM practices reveal how difficult it is to create the randomized, double-blind, controlled studies that are considered the Gold Standard of Western medicine. In a controlled study, everyone in each group is treated exactly the same. As we will learn, the greatest strength of OM is its ability to treat everyone individually. If we are treating everyone the same, we are not practicing Oriental Medicine.

At Pulling Down the Moon, we honor clinical evidence, but choose to also honor empirical evidence, another term for the observed outcomes of clinical practice.

Jeanie writes:

I met Marie just a day after her 40th birthday and she was still getting over the shock that she was turning 40 and did not yet have any children. "This is not how I had planned my life. I thought once I was settled with my career, I'd get married and have a family. I did not think I would have problems since everyone in my family had been fertile," Marie said on our first consultation.

Marie, a financial analyst with a jet-set life, had been married to Don, another financial analyst from the same firm, for about a year. Due to her age, Marie was told by her doctor that she needed to see a fertility specialist right away if she did not get pregnant within three months. After three unsuccessful attempts, Marie and Don were sent to a reproductive endocrinologist's office. After a thorough fertility work-up, the result was not what Marie and Don had anticipated. Marie discovered that her left fallopian tube was blocked and Don had virtually no sperm count. Needless to say, they decided to pursue IVF right away.

On their first IVF cycle, they had three embryos but did not get pregnant. They did a second cycle about two months later where they had five embryos that did not survive to make the day-three embryo transfer (first IVF was day-three embryo transfer as well). Becoming increasingly alarmed, they decided to immediately try another round of IVF, ignoring their RE's suggestion of going the donor egg route. The result of their third IVF was more disappointing than the two previous. This time Marie was not responding to the IVF stimulation hormones so the cycle was cancelled. That's when Marie came to see me.

Recommended by one of her friends, Marie came to see me out of desperation. From our initial consult, I learned that she had once tried acupuncture for neck pain after an automobile accident she had had five years earlier, which had really helped. Due to her previous experience, Marie was very comfortable with acupuncture sessions. I suggested that she try acupuncture combined with herbal therapy for at least one full menstrual cycle before starting another IVF. Marie agreed to one cycle since she felt she could not afford any additional time, given her advanced maternal age. If unsuccessful, she said they'd look into a donor cycle as their RE recommended.

Within her first menstrual cycle with acupuncture and herbal therapy, Marie's response was quite dramatic. Marie lost about eight pounds that she had gained going through IVF cycles. Additionally, her IBS no longer flared up and her migraine headaches became much less frequent. Marie was beginning to get excited about her improved health and started incorporating yoga and meditation into her daily activities. Seeing herself much healthier, Marie decided to wait another menstrual cycle. I recommended to Marie that Don should also be treated for his low sperm count. On his first visit, Don was very curious about where the needles would be placed for his condition. "It's not where you think they'll go," I said. Many men assume the needles will go into the genitals. This is not the case. Don had never tried acupuncture before but he found it very relaxing. He slept through most of his first session.

Marie and Don did not go back to IVF after Marie's second menstrual cycle as she had planned. Since Marie was starting to see some great results, she committed to weekly acupuncture and herbs for six months. Her husband did as well. Their fourth IVF cycle resulted in 11 eggs, of which 9 eggs fertilized. Don's sperm count went up to 7 million from almost nothing and he was able to donate a "fresh" sample instead of the one obtained through biopsy. Due to their age (Don was 43 and Marie 40), pre-implantation genetic diagnosis (PGD) was performed on their embryos. Five days after Marie's egg retrieval, she had three healthy embryos that passed the PGD test with flying colors and they were transferred.

Marie had a positive pregnancy test with twins. Unfortunately, she miscarried one early on but carried the other to term. Today, Marie and Don are proud parents of a healthy baby boy who was born at 9 lbs and 11 oz.

Benefits of Acupuncture

With natural conception, acupuncture can:
- Regulate the menses. *Controlling irregular menstruation can enable couples to better predict the time of ovulation. It is important for a woman to ovulate at the optimal time so that the body is prepared to transport the egg and receive the embryo.*
- Increase the uterine lining. *Acupuncture can increase blood flow to the uterus, resulting in a thicker uterine lining and creating a more hospitable environment for an embryo to implant. We have seen dramatic improvements with acupuncture and herbal therapy in treating thin endometrial lining.*
- Improve sperm. *Separate studies have shown that acupuncture can increase sperm count, sperm motility, and the percentage of sperm that are normal within a given sample (see Appendix D).*
- Prevent miscarriage. *Certain herbal formulas and acupuncture treatments are known to help secure a fetus and prevent a miscarriage. Pre-conception care about 120 days prior is highly recommended.*

Acupuncture and IVF

In conjunction with in-vitro fertilization (IVF), acupuncture may help:
- Regulate hormones. *This is important because a woman's hormone levels must fall within a desired range in order to continue with treatment.*
- Increase the number of follicles and improve the quality of eggs produced. *Obtaining enough good-quality eggs is the most important factor in determining whether or not IVF will be successful.*
- Increase the likelihood of implantation. *As mentioned before with the "German Study," these benefits were obtained using a uniform acupuncture treatment and only two treatments. Some experts suggest that customized, consistent treatment coupled with herbal therapies could improve success rates to 75 percent.*
- Moderate the side effects of hormone therapy. *The medications given during ART are very powerful and can cause unwanted side effects such as hot flashes, irritability, mood swings, and insomnia. Patients who have undergone ART without, and then with, acupuncture report that the side effects were either minimized or eliminated with the use of acupuncture.*
- Relieve stress. *IVF can be a very stressful process. Acupuncture has been shown to increase beta-endorphins (the body's natural feel-good chemical) in the blood.*

When to See a Doctor

While OM and its diagnostic tools can tell us much about a person's imbalance, they cannot tell us everything. Many couples, for a variety of reasons, will choose to utilize Assisted Reproductive Technologies (ART) along with Eastern techniques and wisdom to aid in their conception. In America, holistic medicine is considered alternative medicine, but as we mentioned earlier we prefer the term "integrative." In China, where it is not uncommon to see acupuncture needles used in the intensive care unit along with EKGs and other tools of modern medicine, doctors assert that using *only* Eastern or *only* Western medical systems is like trying to run on one leg—you cover ground, but not very effectively. When the two systems are combined, a clinician is able to run on "two legs" and the healing potential of medicine is improved.

Infertility is defined clinically as an inability to conceive after one year of unprotected sex if under 35 years old, six months if over 35, and three months if over 40. If you meet this criterion, we recommend that you consult a fertility specialist for a fertility screening. This is not to say you will need to use ART, but it is important to rule certain conditions out. The more information you have, the better you will be able to choose which technique, or combination of techniques, is best for you.

Menstrual Cycle and Oriental Medicine

The inner workings of a woman's physiology can be very complex. Fortunately, every month a woman's body gives her clues about the relative health of the reproductive system. In OM, symptoms present during a woman's menstrual cycle can be a window into her internal balance. There can be variations in things like pain before, during or after menstruation and/or ovulation, amount of blood flow, length of bleeding, color of the blood, presence or absence of clots, abnormal bleeding, headaches, mood swings, hot flashes, night sweats, etc.

Most women pay too little attention to what their bodies are showing and telling them during menstrual cycles. All women should be observant of the changes that occur on a monthly basis, and they should be able to describe these changes. It is recommended that if you are seeing an OM practitioner, that you pay attention to and record your menstrual signs and symptoms. This will be very useful in diagnosing your imbalance. More about the menstrual cycle is found in Appendix B.

Medical Interventions

Depending on the results of your fertility screening, your specialist may recommend:

- *Clomid: a drug to stimulate the production of follicles in the ovaries.*
- *IUI (intra-uterine insemination): injecting prepared sperm directly into the uterus using a thin catheter. This bypasses the cervix. This is done around ovulation with or without hormonal stimulation of the ovaries.*
- *IVF (in-vitro fertilization): the ovaries are stimulated using medication to produce many follicles (eggs), and the eggs are removed from the ovaries and combined with sperm in the lab. A few days later, the fertilized eggs (embryos) are then transferred back into the woman's uterus.*

If your reproductive endocrinologist (RE) believes that there is little or no hope of you or your partner producing a viable egg or sperm, then he/she may recommend that you find a donor. Often, the RE can help with this. If the specialist concludes that the anatomy and physiology of your uterus is not able to carry a pregnancy to term, the specialist may recommend that you find a gestational surrogate to carry your biological baby.

Clomid, IUI, and IVF techniques are the most commonly used forms of ART today, but the field of reproductive technology is always evolving and developing more effective techniques. Your RE will know what procedure may be best for you.

Common Causes of Infertility

Several causes of infertility may be classified as ovulatory or pituitary disorders. These include high prolactin level, polycystic ovarian syndrome (PCOS), anovulation, premature ovarian failure, and adrenal and/or pituitary tumors. A history of endometriosis, pelvic inflammatory diseases (with or without history of STDs), adhesions, fibroids, blocked tubes, and abnormal uterine anatomy are all considered anatomical causes of infertility. Recurrent or habitual miscarriage is also considered a form of infertility. For men, sperm production, hormonal imbalance, prior injuries and/or surgeries, history of illness (such as cancer and cancer treatments), and physical abnormalities such as varicoceles are all possible causes.

So, with women, the specialists will be looking to see if there is any problem with the structure, or function of the reproductive system, or with ability to retain a pregnancy. With men, it is mostly a question of their "swimmers." Often, all of this investigation and analysis fails to identify a cause for infertility, thus it is referred to as "unexplained". This is the frustrating "non-diagnosis" that many couples are given.

Rest assured, unexplained infertility is common, and by working with both Eastern and Western approaches there are ways to overcome this diagnosis. In fact, at PDtM we find unexplained infertility is the kind that most positively responds to a blend of holistic and medical fertility treatment.

Fertility Screening

When you meet with your fertility specialist, you and your partner will undergo several tests in an attempt to identify the cause of your difficulty. It will include a thorough history (medical, fertility, sexual) and physical examination of both partners. Blood work will be taken to evaluate hormone levels and glandular functions. For females, blood samples may be taken at several different times in a menstrual cycle, as hormone values fluctuate naturally. Of particular importance are estrogen, FSH (follicle stimulating hormone), LH (luteinizing hormone), progesterone, prolactin, and TSH (thyroid stimulating hormone). See Table 2.1 below for more detail regarding desirable levels. Deviations from the norms in any of these values can significantly impair fertility.

These values may be slightly different from center to center. Also, remember that lab values are not the only thing that's important, and that lab values can change.

In addition to the lab screenings, your specialist will also want to evaluate your physical structures. Pelvic and saline ultrasounds may be used to look for polyps, fibroids, and structural abnormalities. CT and MRI may also be used to better visualize the area. Hysterosalpingogram

TABLE 2.1 FEMALE HORMONE VALUES

HORMONE	DAY TESTED	NORMAL VALUE	INTERPRETATION
E2 (estrogen)	2 or 3	25-75 pg/ml	Too low = ovarian suppression Too high may indicate cysts
FSH (follicle stimulating hormone)	2 or 3	3-20 mIU/ml	<6 best 6-9 good 9-11 borderline >11 possible peri-menopause
LH (luteinizing hormone)	Day 2 or 3 Surge day	< 7 mIU/ml >20 mIU/ml	Too high may indicate PCOS
P4 (progesterone)	Day 2 or 3 7 DPO	<1.5 ng/ml >15 ng/ml	Higher = lower pregnancy rates Indicates ovulation
Prolactin	Day 2 or 3	< 24 ng/m	>24 may interfere w/ ovulation and indicate pituitary tumor or PCOS

(HSG) is a procedure that injects dye into the uterus and uses x-ray to see if the dye can travel through the fallopian tubes. If it can, then the tubes are clear; if it cannot, this suggests possible obstruction in the fallopian tubes. If these techniques are still insufficient, the specialist may look directly into the pelvic cavity via laparoscopy or hysteroscopy (using a small camera to visualize the inside and outside of the uterus, ovaries, and fallopian tubes).

The male must have a semen analysis where the count, motility (how well the sperm move), and morphology (the shape of the sperm) are analyzed. Hormone analysis is also typical. If necessary, a biopsy may be taken of testicular tissue.

Oriental medicine concepts

Oriental Medicine (OM) is based on principles that developed over thousands of years in China. Since what is practiced mostly in present-day America is a combination of techniques that have developed in many Asian countries, we use the term Oriental Medicine, or OM, to describe the techniques of acupuncture, herbs, Asian exercise techniques (tai chi, Qi Gong, etc.), and dietetics to describe this traditional healing system. OM is based on a different understanding of the world. Just as a chemist and a physicist look at the world differently, so does the OM practitioner. The OM view is largely based on observations of nature. It is believed that the way nature works outside the body is the way that it works inside the body. The more we emulate nature, the better off we will be. This section will introduce some of the main concepts of Oriental Medicine.

Yin and Yang

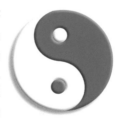

OM is based on Oriental philosophy, which centers on the concept of *balance*. Achieving and maintaining balance is the goal of life. When we are in balance, our bodies and minds should function optimally: the organs should work together properly, sleep should be restful and appropriate, there should be no pain, etc., and a woman who has not yet reached menopause should be able to conceive a child. Oriental Medicine is all about helping restore the body to balance so that it may work the way in which it was intended.

The yin-yang, or Tai Chi symbol, is the classic illustration of the governing principle of Oriental Medicine: balance. The yin-yang theory teaches us to understand all phenomena as lying between two polar extremes. Yang is the lighter, louder, harder, outward, active, masculine aspect of things; while yin is the darker, quieter, softer, inward, restful, and feminine aspect. Neither is better and neither could exist without the other. As you look at the symbol, you will also notice that it is not split evenly in half. As you go around the circle, yang increases until it reaches a maximum, then it starts to wane as yin begins growing, just as the sun reaches its height in the middle of the day and then begins to fall.

It is a dynamic balance. This is the way of nature. The more we learn to accept the cyclical, seasonal nature of life and allow ourselves to step into the flow, the easier we will find it to achieve and maintain balance.

In general, the American lifestyle is very yang. You need to be sure to get some yin time into your schedules. Walking, appreciating art, meditating, practicing Tai Chi, reading for pleasure, listening to music, are all good yin-type activities. We tend to be too focused on "doing;" you should spend more time just "being." And don't forget about sleep. Nighttime is yin time, the time when the body repairs itself. In addition, as you will read in Chapter 4, sleep is also an important part of becoming fully fertile. You are like an Indianapolis race car: you can go very fast, but if you don't make some pit-stops, you'll never finish the race

Jeanie writes: Going with the Flow

Rebecca was a 36-year-old very successful, highly driven career woman who had achieved all the goals she had laid out for herself. So when she had trouble conceiving, she instinctively tried to take control of the situation. Rebecca read as many books as she could on fertility, and she used to call me regularly (at least twice a day, if not more!) to ask what she should do in every little situation. Rebecca was especially inquisitive about what to eat and what not to eat; she once asked me if she should have vinaigrette or ranch dressing since I advised her to minimize dairy (please see Chapter 3, nutrition section, for more detail on dairy consumption). What I had to keep telling her was "stop worrying about what to do in every little situation. This obsession will throw you out of balance more than anything you do in any given situation!" That did not stop her.

After one of her IVF embryo transfers, Rebecca spent five days in "self-imposed bed rest," only getting out of the bed to use the bathroom. Although her doctor told her to just "take it easy," she took this to the extreme. Rebecca went through several unsuccessful IVF cycles. She eventually "down-graded" her ART intervention to monthly IUIs. When she finally relaxed, and gave up her need to control, she finally conceived and had a beautiful baby girl. On the day of her successful IUI, she did not go straight to her usual bed rest. Rather, she went out to enjoy herself, riding roller coasters with her husband since it was their anniversary. I believe it was her releasing of control that allowed her to return to balance.

Qi

A central concept in OM is "Qi." It is like prana, discussed in Chapter 1. Qi (pronounced *chee*) loosely translates as "vital energy" or "life energy." It flows within us and around us, giving all things life, animation, warmth, and form. Similar to electricity, Qi is invisible but its effects

Balance

This idea of balance is also a fundamental concept of the physiology and philosophy of both yoga and its sister science of medicine, Ayurveda. One perfect example of the importance of balance in yoga is the practice of hatha yoga, the yoga practice we learned in Chapter 1. The word "hatha" is an amalgam of two Sanskrit words: ha, which means sun and tha, which means moon. In yoga anatomy there are three major energy channels in the body. The pingala is related to the logical, masculine, and conscious qualities of the sun, and the ida is related to the emotional, feminine, and unconscious qualities of the moon.

Between the ida and the pingala lies the susumna, the central channel. When we are in perfect balance, our energy is believed to be flowing in the susumna, which is neither logical nor emotional, but aligned with pure, spiritual awareness. The practice of hatha yoga is designed to balance the flow of energies between the ida and the pingala, to create optimal physical health, peace of mind, and spiritual awareness. Ayurveda uses the concepts of three gunas—rajas, tamas and sattva—to describe these basic life energies. Rajas is associated with action and change (yang), tamas with inactivity and darkness (yin), and sattva with purity, clarity, and healthy calm (yin-yang balance, or the Tai Chi symbol).

can be seen. When the Qi is flowing in harmony, the body is able to take care of itself. However, the flow of Qi can become obstructed or unbalanced. Acupuncture is the practice of inserting hair-thin needles into the body to affect and re-balance the flow of Qi. As it is written in classical texts, "Where the Qi flows, the Blood goes," so by moving the Qi, we can move the Blood. You can read more about acupuncture later in this chapter.

Jeanie writes:

Many Westerners have difficulty believing in Qi, since it cannot be seen or isolated. I was once at a dinner party and one of the guests who happened to be a medical doctor was doubting the idea of Qi. He said, "If you show me a test tube full of Qi, then I'll believe in it." I said to him, "Okay, but can you show me a test tube full of love, or fear? Do you think these things do not affect our physiology?" He stopped arguing after that.

Blood

As Qi is yang in nature, Blood is yin in nature. Just as the seas must evaporate and fall as rain to feed the rivers and lakes, so too must our circulation be in balance with Qi and Blood. OM's concept of Blood is similar to our understanding in the West: circulation. Blood flows through vessels and nourishes tissues. OM also ascribes the properties of cooling and calming to the function of Blood. For optimal health and fertility, you must have sufficient Blood and it must circulate properly. Acupuncture, herbal therapy, and yoga practice (see Chapter 1) can be effective in improving the Blood flow into the reproductive area.

Fluid and Essence (Jing)

The "Fluid" in OM, also known as "moisture," is another important substance in the body. The Fluid is the substance that lubricates, moistens and nourishes the bodily organs and tissues. Sweat, saliva, vaginal discharge and semen are all forms of Fluids. Too much or too little Fluid can damage proper bodily functions. A simple example can be seen in your bowel movements. Too much or too little moisture can be a problem.

Another concept to introduce is the concept of "essence," which in OM is called "Jing." Jing is your "Youthful Essence" but also your reproductive essence. When we are born, we are full of Jing. But as we live and age we consume it. This is similar to how a candle must burn its wax in order to give light.

Everyone uses up their Jing at different rates. Some deplete their Jing much faster than others; especially those whose lifestyle, diet, and attitudes are our of balance. It is important to live a balanced and moderate lifestyle to conserve your Jing. Lack of Jing can sometimes be seen as premature signs of aging. These include premature graying of the hair, wrinkles, and diminished reproductive capacity. On a daily basis, additional Jing can be acquired through diet, and through exercise such as "Qi Gong." But if you burn through your Jing faster than you can acquire it, you will speed your aging and impair your body's functioning. In Oriental Medicine, acupuncture, herbal therapy and Qi Gong practises are ways to control the consumption of Jing and to help supplement what has been lost.

THE INTERNAL ORGANS

OM ascribes different functionality to the internal organs than we do in the West. So let us be clear that when we discuss them, we are referring to the OM understanding of the organ, and not necessarily the physical organs themselves.

Liver

The Liver is in charge of keeping things flowing smoothly, or "free-coursing," as it is called in OM. Circulation is vital, and the Liver is supposed to ensure that free-flow. OM does not have a strict delineation between the physical, mental, and emotional. Everything that happens in the mind can affect the body and vice-versa.

The Liver has a special relationship with governing emotions because when we get stuck on a feeling, our thoughts stagnate and do not flow freely. Most relationships in OM are both "chicken" and "egg." Impaired circulation can harm the Liver and a weak Liver can impair circulation. When we are depressed, or fearful, or overly joyful, or particularly angry, we can get stuck on those thoughts, causing or displaying stagnation. Our thoughts and emotions should be like the wind: felt when they are here, and gone when the event passes.

The Liver also stores the blood, making it intimately tied to menstruation. It governs the connective tissue. The emotion that can most damage the Liver is anger. Dysfunctions of the Liver can manifest as: migraine headaches, indigestion, bloating, vision problems, tendon problems, cold hands and feet, hypertension, and any type of menstrual problem. Since the Liver is in charge of the sinews, disorders of the Liver can cause erectile dyfunction and sexual impotence in men, and frigidity in women. Again, when we talk about Liver problems in OM, we are not referring to the physical function of the Liver.

Heart

The Heart in OM is considered the Emperor organ. It governs the movement of Blood, but it also houses the mind and spirit. The Heart maintains the proper functioning of all the organs in the system. In OM, the Heart also controls consciousness, intelligence, memory, sleep, and emotions. Fertility is always an emotional journey. These strong emotions can tax the Heart. This is why you need to minimize your stress in order to maximize your fertility.

Since the Heart has the aspect of fire element in OM theory, imbalance can cause the organ to overheat. This can manifest as dry mouth and thirst (especially at night), cold sore and/or canker sores, anxiety, agitation, insomnia, and nightmares. Ironically, the emotion that can damage the Heart is Joy. While happiness is a good and desirable thing, it too must be in balance. In OM, it is interpreted that an over-abundance of Joy can cause "manic" behaviors in people.

Meditation, which has been gaining popularity in the West, has been practiced in Asia for thousands of years. The philosophy behind meditation is to empty the "mind" (sections 2 and 3 of this book will delve deeper into this concept). This is practiced so that the Heart, which houses both mind and spirit, can rest itself. When the mind is always in motion, the Heart Spirit cannot rest. It is said in Asian philosophy that when the mind is empty, the Heart can truly open to receiving its Spirit, the unconditional love that heals all things. Libido belongs to the activity of the Spirit, since it is believed in OM that all human desires are related to the Spirit.

You can practice strengthening the Heart by practicing smiling. Smile in front of the mirror; make sure you're smiling from the bottom of your Heart! Let yourself feel happy. This true smiling can have a positive effect not only on your Heart, but on your whole body: physically, mentally, and spiritually.

Spleen

The main purpose of the Spleen is to control and maintain the proper functioning of digestion. The Spleen, paired with the Stomach, processes the food and turns it into the Qi, Blood and Jing (Essence) that we use for daily activities. Improper diet and/or poor eating habits, prolonged exposure to dampness (internally or externally), over-thinking, or pensiveness, can damage the Spleen and Stomach. Since all functions depend on Qi, Blood and Jing, maintaining a healthy Spleen and Stomach is very important. You must examine and adjust your diet to protect your Spleen. Please see the Nutrition section of Chapter 3 for more information about a Fully Fertile diet.

The impaired function of Spleen and Stomach can lead to digestive problems, poor appetite, diarrhea, allergies, anemia, chronic fatigue, easy bruising, cold and sweaty hands and feet, headaches, obesity, and problems with menstrual bleeding.

Lung

The Lung, with its position at the top of the organ system according to OM, has the important function of forming and distributing the Qi. As we breathe, the Lung forms the life energy Qi with the breath we take and sends the Qi through the body to moisten, protect, and nourish the body.

The Lung, being the umbrella of the other organs, is usually the first to be affected by invading pathogens. It governs the Fluid distribution which includes controlling the pores and maintaining the skin. The disorders in the Lung can give rise to dry, itchy skin, rashes, shortness of breath, abnormal sweating, respiratory problems, diarrhea or constipation, edema, and fatigue. The Lung can easily be damaged by excessive grief.

Kidney

In OM the Kidney is probably the most important organ for reproduction. The Kidney also stores the Jing, which is our youthful essence and our reproductive essence. To work on the Jing we must work on the Kidneys.

Excessive exercise, over-consumption of cold and raw foods, and many nights of missed sleep in order to finish work, can significantly damage the Jing. This is detrimental to fertility since the Kidney essence declines naturally, and the decline is accelerated by these lifestyle choices. So don't burn yourself out! The Kidney is considered the "root" organ. Kidney Yin is the root of all yin, and Kidney Yang is the root of all yang; so a deficiency in yin or yang may be treated through the kidneys. It is the water organ and controls water metabolism, elimination, and sexual activity. It is most affected by fright (the way fear can cause one's urine to descend). Nuts and seeds, marrow, and shellfish are considered good Kidney foods in OM.

Tools and Techniques of Oriental Medicine

Four Examinations

So, how can OM diagnose your imbalance? OM practitioners use a traditional method of diagnosis called the Four Examinations. They are: looking, feeling, asking questions, and smelling. While this may sound simplistic, a practitioner will evaluate your overall presentation, quality of voice, word choice, body language, body type, skin, pulse, color, texture, and shape of the tongue. An OM practitioner will ask about many areas of your functioning; from digestion to sleep to mood, appetite, circulation, and respiration, many of which may seem to be unrelated to the reasons you're seeking treatment.

One of the most important aspects of diagnosing infertility in OM is extensive questioning about women's menstrual cycle, discharges, pregnancies, miscarriages, and childbirth(s). A well-trained OM practitioner can tell a lot about a woman by her menstrual history. Most commonly asked questions regarding menstrual cycle include: cycle length, amount of blood flow, color of the blood, quality (such as clotty discharge), and pain associated with the menstrual cycle. Pregnancy and miscarriage history can also be very useful in determining one's constitution or imbalances. Once a condition or pattern has been diagnosed, OM has tools to help correct the imbalance, including exercises like Qi Gong, and treatments such as acupuncture and herbal therapy.

Qi Gong

Qi in "Qi Gong" is same as the word Qi described earlier in this chapter; Gong means "work" or "practice." Qi Gongis a holistic healing method involving postures, movements, breathing, and meditation to heal and maintain harmony and balance within the body. In the Chinese ideogram, the character represents air and food. Air that we breathe, and the food that we consume, all turn into Qi in our bodies. Qi Gong is as much about what is going on in the spirit and mind as it is what you are doing with your body. Daily practice helps bring the mind into a state of tranquility and fine tunes the body. Unlike tai chi, Qi Gong is also used as a medical art, to heal oneself or others.

Just like yoga, Qi Gong has been practiced in China and many other Asian countries for thousands of years. It is one of the most portable, yet effective ways to restore health. In Qi Gong, there are three important energy centers or elixir fields in the body: lower Dan Tien, middle Dan Tien and upper Dan Tien. The lower Dan Tien is located between the navel and the pubic bone (around the second chakra in yoga), otherwise known as the "core" in the West. This is known as the root, where the energy is cultivated to fuel the whole body. The middle Dan Tien is by the solar plexus, and governs mostly digestion and respiration.

The upper Dan Tien is between the two eyebrows, also known as the Third eye. It is the center of our consciousness and houses the spirit.

In Qi Gong, lower Dan Tien is the most emphasized area of the three Dan Tiens. It is the energy center that must be strong to sustain everything else in the body. It is the root of our sexual energy, the most primordial energy of human life. This is also where the conception and the growth of the fetus occurs in women. One of the most basic exercises for cultivating this area is "abdominal breathing." It is also known as natural breathing, and we are all born to breathe this way.

Physiologically, this type of breathing is much more effective than breathing with our chest, as most people often do. When we breathe into our abdomen, the diaphragm lowers, creating more room for the lungs to expand. Whether we realize it or not, breathing regulates pH: inhaling brings alkaline oxygen into the system, and exhaling removes acidic carbon dioxide. When we breathe shallowly, into our chest, it increases the acidity of our blood. Breathing into the lower abdomen also helps balance the pH in the body and energizes the lower Dan Tien. While most of us do not often think about how we are breathing, the consequences can be profound.

WEEK 2 ACTIVITY 1: NATURAL BREATHING EXERCISE

Here's a simple breathing exercise that can help to cultivate our lower "Dan Tien," our core. In this exercise, inhale through the nose and exhale through the mouth. Our nose serves to filter out the impurities, so make sure to breathe in through the nose whenever possible. When practicing this breathing exercise, wear comfortable clothes and remove all jewelry. Sit in a chair comfortably, but do not lean on the backrest. As you slowly inhale, expand your abdomen and lower back. You can place your hands on the abdomen and on your back to feel the breath filling this area of the body.

At the end of the inhalation, hold your breath for a second and be aware of this moment. This is the moment that inhalation changes to exhalation. In OM, this is the moment that changes from yin (inhalation) to yang (exhalation). Exhale slowly and breathe out all the air in the abdomen and the lower back through the mouth. Repeat for five to ten minutes.

This breathing can be incorporated at any time of the day. If you feel stressed, or tired, rest for a few minutes and try this breathing. You can also try this breathing if you have a hard time falling asleep. This is an effective way to create awareness of your body and give it 100 percent of the attention that it deserves.

ACUPUNCTURE

So what is acupuncture? How does it work? How can it help with fertility? Western science has tried to understand acupuncture in Western terms. It has been postulated that it works on the nervous system, endocrine system, lymphatic system, etc; but all of these explanations have proven insufficient.

Over the past 4,000 years, Asian physicians have mapped the flow of Qi in the body and have determined that it flows through 14 main channels. Each channel connects with, and is named for, an internal organ. They are Lung, Large Intestine, Stomach, Spleen, Heart, Small intestine, Urinary bladder, Kidney, Pericardium, Triple Warmer, Gallbladder, and Liver. Among these, Triple Warmer is the only one that does not correspond to a single physical structure. Rather, it describes three cavities of the torso namely, the pleural (Lung), abdominal, and pelvic cavities. Together, these channels are known as the meridian system. The Qi flows throughout the body from one meridian to the next in a closed circuit.

There are also smaller capillary vessels that carry the Qi to every cell in the body. It is believed that the meridian system is the most primitive and basic system of communication in the body, and that even when we were eight-celled embryos, those cells communicated with each other through Qi. As we developed, other physiological systems such as skeletal, muscular, circulatory, nervous, etc. continued to expand on this foundation. When Qi flows harmoniously, the body functions optimally. However, the flow of Qi can become obstructed or unbalanced, causing disruption in the other, higher systems. Acupuncture utilizes the influential points (such as the acupuncture points, found through years of experimentation) on the meridians to bring Qi back into balance. When the foundation is stable, all that is built upon it will work better.

There are different ways to understand the meridian system. One likens it to a series of rivers. The rivers get blocked and the acupuncture needles remove the obstruction. Another way to look at it is like a circuit board. Inserting needles throws the switches to re-direct the flow of energy. Western science has trouble accepting this system because the meridians and Qi cannot be seen. Interesting research using Western medical imaging techniques is beginning to demonstrate the existence of this system. Even in China, there's still some disagreement over how acupuncture really works

Acupuncture Treatments

Acupuncture treatment is preceded by a thorough evaluation by your practitioner. After determining the imbalance, your practitioner will insert anywhere between 5–20 acupuncture needles into acupuncture points selected. Then you will lie comfortably in a dark room with aromatherapy and soft music or guided meditation. Some practitioners prefer to leave their patients alone with their thoughts.

During this time, most patients experience a state of deep relaxation. Sometimes, depending on the presenting symptoms of the patients, traditional techniques such as cupping, moxibustion (burning of small amount of herb called mugwort, artemisia vulgaris over acupuncture points), and electro-stimulation can be incorporated in the course of treatment. The whole procedure usually takes less than one hour. After a treatment, you will be fine to return to all your daily activities.

Nobody likes the idea of needles. But not all needles are created equal. Acupuncture needles are extremely thin and can often penetrate the skin with no pain at all. Some areas may be more sensitive and feel like a small pinch as the needle is inserted, but this sensation generally subsides within a few seconds. Once the needles are in place, most people do not feel anything at all. Sometimes, a light, tingling, buzz-like sensation can be felt with warmth around the needle insertion point. Other times people feel a sensation of cool running through their meridian channels. Other descriptions of the sensation accompanying acupuncture treatment vary widely—from actually feeling the movement of Qi to feeling nothing at all.

Acupuncture and Male Factor Issues

Infertility with male factor issues can be frustrating, and couples may wonder what can be done. Unfortunately, Western medicine offers very few options when dealing with this problem. On the other hand, acupuncture has shown promising results on male infertility. Research has shown that men who receive acupuncture treatments have an increased sperm count, improved sperm motility, and higher percental of "normal" sperm in a given ejaculate (see Apendix D for more informtion on this research) This is how acupuncture can help at the physical level. It also works on an energetic level: we find the couples who walk the path together tend to have better results.

The Tai Chi symbol from the earlier section represents the unity between yin and yang. Yin represents the female and the yang represents the male; yin cannot exist without yang or vice versa. As we all know, it takes two to make the baby. All the best treatments and care in the world can be given to either a woman or a man, but it will still be only 50 percent of the whole. One cannot donate 50 percent of sperm or 50 percent of the egg to create a life. It must be 100 percent complete; hence, both women and men should be treated.

A sperm cycle, from generation to full maturation, takes about 90 days. It is optimal for men to start acupuncture treatments about 3 months or 90 days prior to sperm donation; especially for males with known sperm issues.

HERBAL THERAPY

It should come as no surprise that plants and animal materials can have effects on the body. Everything under the sun has properties: some are warming, some cooling, some activating, some sedating, etc. To give you an example, think of the times when you put a piece of mint leaf in your mouth and a dab of cinnamon. You probably felt the cooling sensation with the mint leaf and a bit of warm and spicy sensation with the cinnamon. In herbalism, mint is used to induce a cooling effect on the body such as reducing fever, and cinnamon is used to warm a chilled body, like when you're just catching cold. The Chinese have been observing and documenting these effects for thousands of years. One of the earliest written herbal therapy texts dates back to China more that two thousand years ago. There, and in many other Asian countries, herbal therapy is the primary mode of treating illness.

In Oriental herbal therapy, just like acupuncture, the illness and/or disorder are diagnosed according to individual patterns using the examinations described earlier in this chapter. By properly combining herbs, a skilled herbalist can create a formula that addresses the patient's imbalance completely and accurately. In herbal medicine, it is understood that if a formula causes unwanted side effects, it is clearly not the right formula. Herbal medicines can be customized for each patient's needs and changed gradually as the patient's condition improves. In OM, the herbs are rarely given individually; they are combined with other herbs and minerals according to a patient's specific pattern in order to eliminate unwanted side effects. This is very different from Western medicine. In the Western approach, a drug will be a good match for some, and a fair or poor match for some others. As you may know you cannot put a patent on a plant. That's why many Western medications are actually synthetic versions of plants found in nature. Yes, that's right. The active ingredient in many of the pills we commonly take are synthetic copies of medicines first discovered and tested by herbalists, shamans and traditional healers.

OM is extremely individualized. Every symptom an individual presents with can come from at least two different imbalances. For example, constipation can be caused by too much heat in the body. Heat dries the stool and makes it hard to pass. But constipation may also be caused by too much cold in the body. Cold makes things tighten up and stop moving. Herbs that cool the digestive track will help the hot-type constipation, but will make a person with cold-type constipation worse. Similar symptoms may require different treatments. For this reason, people should not take herbs or supplements without proper guidance. Similarly, the same imbalance (such as too much heat) can manifest in different ways in different people (constipation, hypertension, eczema, etc.) OM uses its system of diagnosis to look past the symptom to identify the underlying cause.

Most of the few incidents of herb toxicities and herb-drug interactions are caused by self-prescribing or friends recommending herbs. Very few herbs are good for a condition, most are good for a condition *when caused* by a particular imbalance. There is no herb for upset stomach, but there are herbs for upset stomach due to deficient Spleen Qi, or due to damp accumulating in the stomach, or to over-consumption of meat, or due to blood stasis, etc. One must identify the pattern of imbalance before selecting the treatment, not just one symptom. This requires training.

Herbs for Fertility

In regards to fertility and herbal therapy, there are a great many herbs that can help. But again, they must be correctly prescribed according to your particular pattern, not just your diagnosis. Oriental herbal therapy has some of its roots in Taoism, which is an Eastern philosophy. The goal in Taoism is to go with the natural flow of the universe, and by correct action and thought (or inaction and lack-of-thought), one can achieve immortality. In their quest, the Chinese Taoist herbalists found many herbs that increase longevity and restore youthfulness. It should be no surprise that some of the herbs that restore youthfulness can also restore or improve reproductivity. In addition, there are herbs and formulas that help all the things acupuncture can help (regulating menses, building endometrium, treating fibroids and endometriosis, preventing miscarriage, etc.) Herbal therapies have been utilized in helping couples achieve pregnancy for thousands of years for one simple reason: it works. However, in the modern day with new medications and the very precise micromanagement of a woman's physiology in an ART cycle, many REs prefer that patients do not use any herbs or supplements while undergoing stimulation. While we do not feel that it is harmful, it is true that we do not know the effects of combining our time-tested herbal therapies with the newest pharmaceutical treatments. You should discuss this topic with your acupuncturist and your reproductive endocrinologist to ensure the best course of treatment.

At Pulling Down the Moon, practitioners incorporate herbal therapy whenever appropriate and possible. Our experience has shown that using herbal therapy when patients are not undergoing any hormone stimulation such as IVF or IUI, improved patients' overall clinical response. Women produced more and better-quality eggs, had fewer side effects from the hormone stimulation, and had higher rates of achieving and maintaining pregnancy. Again, if you are interested in using herbal therapy, be sure to discuss it thoroughly with your practitioners and physicians before you start. As much as something can help in the right circumstances, it can be detrimental in the wrong ones. To find a qualified practitioner near you, please refer to the Find Practitioners page of Appendix A.

Jeanie writes:

Sandra came to see me just after a second unsuccessful IVF cycle. Her reproductive endocrinologist (RE) told her that she was a poor IVF responder despite her "normal" hormone levels. Her RE also told her that she could try again, but he was doubtful the cycle would work unless she pursued the donor route. Sandra was not ready to hear that, at the age of 38, she may not be able to get pregnant using her own eggs. She had a four-year-old daughter whom she conceived naturally and she was not ready to give up trying to have another biological child.

I will never forget our first session. Sandra had never tried acupuncture or herbal therapy before and she was a bit nervous during her first session about the "needles." I was not surprised since many people express fear about their first visit and the thought of being poked with needles and looking like a porcupine. I used a dab of lavender oil and worked her through some breathing exercises to induce relaxation. Once she was feeling more comfortable and looking more relaxed, I decided to start the acupuncture session. As soon as I told her that I would now be putting the needles in her, she sat straight up.

"Are you sure this doesn't hurt?" she asked, now reversing all the relaxation work we had just completed for the last 15 minutes. I asked her to give me one of her hands and I pinched it. "Did that hurt?" I asked. She replied, "No." "That's what most of the needle insertions will feel like," I said.

"Really, that's it, are you sure?" She questioned with an expression that showed both relief and disbelief.

"Yes, for the most part," I answered. Sandra lay back down. She was breathing rapidly so I went through the breathing exercise again with her. Within a few breaths, I could see her calming down again.

As I wiped the acupuncture points with the alcohol wipes, she yelled out "Thirteen!?"

"Thirteen? What do you mean?" I asked.

"You just wiped thirteen places. Is that where you are putting the needles?" She questioned in a distraught voice. I never had anyone count before so I was a bit amused.

"Yes, those are the points," I replied with a smile.

"Then do one more or one less, thirteen doesn't seem like a lucky number, especially on my first acupuncture session." Sandra was insistent so I granted her wish and put in fourteen acupuncture needles. She liked the number fourteen because it was two sevens.

To her surprise, Sandra found acupuncture very relaxing. After her first session she said, "Massage feels great afterwards, but acupuncture, boy, it made me melt into the table." She admitted her own anticipation was much worse than the actual treatment. After the first session, the rest was a breeze for her. Rain or shine, Sandra came weekly or sometimes twice a week to have her acupuncture treatments and herbal therapy.

TABLE 2.3 EXAMPLE OF A DAILY ACTIVITY CHART

Qi Drain	Qi Gain
e.g. Not enough sleep	e.g. Yoga

As the weeks went by, Sandra noticed changes in her menstrual cycle. She used to cycle every 31 to 32 days with ovulation around day 17 and 18. By the fourth cycle, Sandra's cycle became much more regular with ovulation occurring around day 14 and menstruation at day 28. Sandra also changed her diet after seeing our nutritionist and took our fertility yoga class. After four months, Sandra became pregnant without assisted reproductive technology and had a healthy, biological, baby boy nine months later.

WEEK TWO ACTIVITY 2: QI GAIN/QI DRAIN

This exercise will help you understand our relationship with Qi. Most of your daily activities deplete Qi. Working, playing, worrying, and exercising all cost us some Qi. We develop or cultivate our Qi by eating nutritious, well-cooked foods, meditating, practicing Tai Chi or yoga, walking for pleasure, appreciating art and music, and other types of restorative activities or non-activities. This can also be thought of in terms of yin and yang. Yang activities are the things that cost us Qi, while yin activities (non-activities) replenish the Qi.

So here is the exercise. Make a list of the various activities in your daily life. Put them into two categories, Qi gain on one side of the paper, Qi drain on the other. You can use the table below to start this. Look at just how many things you do every day that deplete your Qi and how few things you do to restore it. For many of us, this ratio is far from balanced. Since Qi fuels all bodily activities, chronic depletion of Qi will negatively impact our functioning including fertility.

We introduce this concept of balance to many of our patients in this way. We are socialized to always be "doing." We are told, "Don't waste a minute," or "time is precious" or "if you're not getting ahead, you're falling behind," all our lives. We are told that we need to always be productive and are not taught the value in restoration. If you have a greenhouse, you do not leave the grow lights on 24 hours a day. Plants need the yin time to enable them to grow in the next yang phase. Similarly, we need yin time to restore expended Qi and to prepare our bodies and minds for future growth and development. Look at your chart and see how balanced yin and yang are in your daily life. See if there is some room to make adjustments and make your daily routine more balanced.

A Fertility Acupuncture Consultation with Jeanie Lee Bussell

Acupuncture Treatments for IVF Cycles

- *It is never too early to start treatment. In Oriental Medicine, the longer a problem has existed, the longer it takes to correct. The sooner we start getting the body back into balance, the easier it will be and the sooner you will have increased fertility.*
- *Optimally, you should start acupuncture treatments at least three months prior to ART (both male and female). This is the preparatory period. Follicle maturation begins about 120 days before ovulation (see Appendix C, under Ovaries, for more information on egg selection and maturation). It takes about 90 days for sperm to fully mature.*
- *Healthy mind and body = healthy egg and sperm = healthy embryo = healthy pregnancy = healthy child.*
- *During the preparatory period, I recommend acupuncture treatments once or twice a week, depending on the amount of time you have before you start your ART cycle (e.g. if you allow yourself about three months before starting IVF, acupuncture treatments once a week will be sufficient until IVF stimulation begins). If you are starting during the birth control phase, about three to four weeks prior to IVF stimulation, I recommend twice a week until the stimulation.*
- *Once IVF stimulation begins, I recommend at least three to four acupuncture treatments between the start of your FSH (Gonal-F, Follistim, etc.) injections and egg retrieval, based upon your progress. If your response to the hormone stimulation is too fast or too slow (developing too many or too few follicles) you may benefit from more acupuncture treatments. In rare cases, people may benefit most from daily treatment.*
- *After the egg retrieval, once you are comfortably able to, it is a good idea to have an acupuncture treatment to minimize the bloating, distention, and cramping. It also helps better prepare the uterus for implantation.*
- *On a day-three embryo transfer, I recommend two treatments: one before and one after the transfer. Studies have shown that this protocol significantly increase pregnancy rates (see Appendix D). If you are having a day-five embryo transfer, I recommend one acupuncture treatment before or after the embryo transfer (if you'd like to do before and after, that would still be fine. There are currently no studies done with day-five embryo transfer, but from our clinical experience, we have seen an increase in pregnancy rates with incorporating acupuncture treatment on day five as well.)*
- *Follow up with an acupuncture treatment about five to seven days after the transfer.*
- *Once you have a positive pregnancy test, I recommend acupuncture once a week, through the first trimester (when miscarriage is most likely to occur).*
- *If there are any symptoms associated with pregnancy such as morning sickness, bleeding, or pain, you may need to be seen more frequently.*

Acupuncture Treatments During IUI (Intrauterine Insemination) Cycle

- Preparation before starting an IUI cycle is the same as for an IVF cycle (see Acupuncture Treatments for IVF Cycles).
- During the follicle stimulation, whether it's clomid, injectables or natural (no artificial stimulation), two to three acupuncture treatments until the trigger shot (hCG injection) is recommended.
- You should have one acupuncture treatment before or after IUI; preferably on the day of the IUI.
- One follow-up acupuncture treatment 7–10 days after the IUI.
- Once you have a positive pregnancy test, the treatment recommendation is the same as for IVF (opposite).

Donor Egg Cycle or Frozen Embryo Transfer

- Again, I generally recommend one acupuncture treatment per week until embryo transfer.
- On the day of the embryo transfer, I suggest an acupuncture treatment before and after.
- One follow-up acupuncture treatment about 7 days after the embryo transfer.

Preparation for Men

- Regardless of the cause of infertility, I recommend that both partners be treated. It works on a biochemical level by improving their body's functioning, but it also seems to work on an energetic level: couples who walk the path together tend to fare better than those who walk it alone.
- As I have mentioned before, it takes about 90 days for the sperm to reach maturity. Males with no known pathology should be treated on a weekly basis until sperm is collected for use, preferably beginning at least three months prior to the planned cycle. For males with known issues, I highly recommend that they start acupuncture treatment as early as possible. We have seen improvements in all sperm parameters (count, motility, and morphology), both in our own clinical practice and in clinical research studies.
- If possible, the male partner should try to have an acupuncture treatment a day before sperm donation.

Fully Fertile Diet

THE FIRST THING we have to say about fertility nutrition is that a whole book could be, and several have been, written on this topic and we highly recommend that you read them. If you do, one thing you'll notice is that there is as yet very little consensus about what makes a diet a "fertility diet." This is primarily because the clinical data needed to make definitive recommendations regarding optimal dietary composition and the best and worst foods for fertility is incomplete. In most cases, nutritionists are forced to make "best practice" guidelines based on studies that measure hormone levels instead of pregnancy outcomes or are in some other way one step removed from the question at hand: will this diet help a woman get pregnant?

Sure, some studies show that diets high in soy protein lower the levels of important ovarian hormones, but others indicate that women in Asia, where the diet is higher in soy, do not have higher rates of infertility than in the US. Data from the National Nurses' Study II is confusing on the topic of dairy. One finding shows the intake of low-fat dairy was associated with higher rates of ovulatory infertility, another finding from the same study showed that eating ice cream seemed to protect against infertility. There's a growing body of evidence suggesting that lower carbohydrate diets, where the intake of carbohydrate is about 40 percent of total calories, is effective at improving glucose metabolism and ovarian hormone levels in patients with Polycystic Ovarian Syndrome (PCOS). But do these women conceive at a higher rate than women who achieve blood sugar control through a diet that is less restrictive of carbohydrates but focuses on eliminating highly processed grains and refined sugars? Alas, we simply do not yet know the answers to these important questions.

The very nature of the fertility journey—the urgency, the sense of a ticking clock, the emotional roller coaster—makes waiting the year or more it would take to obtain good, prospective research studies into the link between diet and fertility seem untenable.

Nevertheless, it also does not mean we should rush to judgment or go off the "nutrition deep-end" with highly restrictive diets. But don't despair. If we managed to sum up the teachings of Oriental Medicine in the last chapter, we believe we can hit the highlights of fertility nutrition here. Although the guidelines we will present in this chapter just scratch the surface of a rich vein of information about diet and fertility, we know they are valuable because we see the wisdom of these recommendations at work in our patients. Many of these patients have improved their menstrual function, responded better to fertility treatment, and eventually become pregnant by implementing these guidelines. In addition, you will find that these recommendations also agree with OM Dietary Therapy so they will fit seamlessly into your integrative care for fertility program. So hold on to your hats, ladies, here is the recipe for fertility-friendly eating *à la* PDtM.

Components of the Fully Fertile Diet

Did you realize that your ovaries are acutely aware of what you eat, when you eat, and how much you eat? And we're not just talking in a general "you are what you eat" way. We're talking an immediate, minute-to-minute kind of way. Many of us think of ovaries as little sacs that simply incubate and release eggs each month, but they're actually incredibly sensitive and complex endocrine organs, designed to receive and broadcast hormonal signals that make our reproductive system the amazing symphony of creation that it is.

Scientists call the communication between the ovaries and the master endocrine glands of the brain, hypothalamus, and pituitary, the *hypothalamic-pituitary-ovarian axis*, or the HPO axis, and it functions like a feedback loop. The major hormone signals for reproduction come from the pituitary gland via the hormones FSH (follicle stimulating hormone) and LH (leutinizing hormone). These hormones attach to receptor proteins in the ovarian cells at different points in the menstrual cycle and tell the ovaries to send out the hormonal signals (estrogen, progesterone, and other androgens) that regulate the menstrual cycle. In return, signals from the developing ovarian follicles "feed back" to tell the brain to either increase or decrease FSH and LH. When all hormones are present at their appropriate levels during the different phases of the menstrual cycle, healthy egg development and ovulation occurs. This "conversation" between ovaries and brain takes place via the blood stream, in the presence of many other hormones including cortisol (stress hormone), hormones and chemicals from food sources (soy isoflavones, hormones from food supply), and our own metabolic hormones.

Stressors

Our hormonal systems are generally resilient to daily stressors. However, when stressors become severe or chronic, disruption of hormonal balance can occur. Lifestyle factors that can impair hormone balance are being overweight, bad nutrition habits, stress and poor sleep quality. In the case of diet, the major culprits are carrying excess weight, eating too much sugar and bad fats and added hormones and chemicals in the food supply—all of which we'll discuss in greater detail in this chapter.

This is not just about women, either. Sperm are also sensitive to nutrition, but in a slightly different way from the ovaries. Unlike a woman's egg cells, which have been present in her ovaries since she was just a fetus in her mom's tummy, a man's sperm begin to form during adolescence from "parent cells" in the lining of his seminiferous tubules. On the way to maturity these primitive cells, called spermatagonia, mature into primary spermatocytes, which then divide twice more to become spermatozoa (sperm) as we know it. Much smaller than the egg, with a tail that's built for movement and a head filled with genetic material, these spermatozoa basically serve as DNA torpedoes. Because of the large amount of cell division involved in the growth and development of sperm, these guys are particularly susceptible to oxidative damage from free radicals (byproducts of oxygen metabolism that cause damage to DNA and cell membranes). Cutting back on toxicity, including smoking, limiting junk food and alcohol, and increasing dietary intake of antioxidant vitamins, can be beneficial to sperm quality.

From this perspective, it's not surprising we believe that the nutritional status of both a woman and her partner is a critical part of their ability to produce healthy eggs and sperm, as well as to sustain a healthy pregnancy. This week you'll learn seven steps you can take toward making your diet "fully fertile," and keep a food journal for one week to see if your current food choices support, rather than sabotage, your reproductive health.

Seven Steps for a Fully Fertile Diet

STEP 1. MAINTAINING YOUR FERTILE WEIGHT

Women who are overweight or obese are at a greater risk of infertility. (*Gesink Law,* 2007) Clinical research also suggests this is true for men. (*Sallman,* 2006)

The American Society for Reproductive Medicine asserts that 12 percent of infertility results from abnormal body weight (6 percent from over, and 6 percent from underweight), and, most surprisingly, more than 70 percent of women who are infertile as a result of body weight disorders will conceive spontaneously if their weight disorder is corrected by a weight-gain or weight-loss program.

What is it about weight that affects our ability to conceive? In the case of women, the main mechanism in the disruption of fertility is believed to be the role that the body's fat cells play in the manufacturing and storage of estradiol, the primary female reproductive hormone. When body fat levels are high, the net result is an excess level of estrogen and its chemical relatives and that hormonal imbalance throws off the reproductive system. In the case of underweight, low levels of body fat mean less circulating estradiol and a gradual down-regulating of the reproductive cycle until it is turned off completely. Everyone is familiar with the amenorrheic athlete and this refers back to the concept of energy balance we discussed at the end of Week 1.

The hormone insulin, which is often elevated in the body of overweight women, can also act directly on the ovaries. Insulin's primary role in the body is to allow the body to store excess blood sugar in fat cells. In overweight women, increased insulin may be produced to regulate higher blood sugar levels. Because insulin is chemically similar to the ovarian hormones which help the eggs mature, the ovaries confuse the elevated insulin with their own growth factors and down-regulate the production of reproductive hormones. In addition, excess levels of insulin can cause certain cells in the ovaries to begin to produce excess androgens, which throw off hormonal balance and can have other negative health consequences, including cosmetic issues like acne, hirsutism, and changes in blood lipid profiles. Insulin also blocks the enzymes that rupture the follicle wall at the time of ovulation. Insulin levels respond to dietary signals so a "fertility diet" for overweight women would seek to normalize blood sugar by cutting back on sweets and simple carbohydrates so lower levels of insulin are needed to process meals. In addition, losing weight also increases the body's insulin sensitivity.

In order to categorize the relationship between weight and infertility, physicians use something called Body Mass Index, or BMI, to estimate a woman's weight-based risk for infertility. Women who fall into the BMI categories of overweight, obese, and extremely

Body Mass Index (BMI)

BMI is determined by converting your weight into kilograms and dividing it by your height in meters squared.

BMI of 19-24 = Healthy
BMI 25-29 = Overweight
BMI 30-39 = Obese
BMI 40+ = Extremely obese

Studies have shown that overweight women (BMI 25 or over) are more likely to have ovulation problems that result in irregular or infrequent menstrual cycles and infertility. Obesity also increases the risk for ectopic pregnancies and miscarriage. With medical fertility treatment, success rates are lower in women who are overweight. Suboptimal response to ART may result from the reduced efficacy of fertility medications and the higher percentage of immature eggs seen in obese women.

obese all have lower pregnancy rates than women with healthy BMIs. Women with BMIs of under 18 are also at higher risk of infertility.

Polycystic Ovarian Syndrome (PCOS)

Any discussion of weight and fertility needs to touch upon the topic of Polycystic Ovarian Syndrome, or PCOS. This disorder of the endocrine system causes disruption of the menstrual cycle. This disorder occurs in about 5–10 percent of women and is associated with a lack of regular ovulation and high levels or activity of androgenic hormones. PCOS is also highly correlated with insulin-resistance and often, but not always, with overweight.

Symptoms of PCOS include irregular or infrequent menstrual periods, infertility related to non-ovulatory cycles, elevated levels of male hormones and abdominal adiposity (the tendency to gain weight around the middle rather than in the hips). Your OB or Reproductive Endocrinologist can diagnose PCOS using a number of different tests including pelvic ultrasound and hormone levels (LH/FSH ratio, circulating testosterone, glucose tolerance testing). Women with PCOS who are trying to conceive are often given Metformin, an oral anti-diabetic drug, and counseled to lose weight (if appropriate) and to use diet and exercise to control their blood sugar levels.

Using BMI to Guide You to Your Fertile Weight

To determine whether you're at your optimal fertile weight, you need to calculate your BMI (see Table 3.1). If your BMI is greater than 18 and lower than 25, you are in the range of your fertile weight. If you have a BMI of 25 and above, determine your goal weight for fertility by following the row of your height in inches over to the BMI column for 24. If your BMI is lower than 19, track the row of your height over to BMI of 19 and find your fertile weight. For example, Susie Q is 5 ft 3 and weighs 176 lbs. To find her BMI, she would cross-reference height in inches (63) with her weight on the chart on page 95. According to the chart, Susie's BMI is 31 and we know that for optimal fertility Susie's BMI should be under 25. To find her fertile weight, she can now cross-reference her height with a BMI of 24 and look at the associated weight. Susie's fertile weight is 135 lbs, so her weight loss goal for fertility would be to lose 41 pounds.

Our fertile weight may be very different from our "desired" body weight. Susie may dream of eventually fitting into a size 6 and weighing 125 pounds. For fertility, however, our goals are based on achieving a weight that is optimal for conception. In general, our fertile weight is more realistic, and therefore easier to maintain, than our "size four fantasies." Nevertheless, with continued healthy eating and a good fitness regimen, Susie may eventually reach her ideal body weight—once her baby is born! But also note, the American Society for Reproductive Medicine (ASRM) suggests that as little as a 10 percent decrease

TABLE 3.1 BODY MASS INDEX MEASUREMENTS

BMI (Height in inches)	Normal						Overweight					Obese										Extreme Obesity														
	19	20	21	22	23	24	25	26	27	28	29	30	31	32	33	34	35	36	37	38	39	40	41	42	43	44	45	46	47	48	49	50	51	52	53	54
												Body Weight (pounds)																								
58	91	96	100	105	110	115	119	124	129	134	138	143	148	153	158	162	167	172	177	181	186	191	196	201	205	210	215	220	224	229	234	239	244	248	253	258
59	94	99	104	109	114	119	124	128	133	138	143	148	153	158	163	168	173	178	183	188	193	198	203	208	212	217	222	227	232	237	242	247	252	257	262	267
60	97	102	107	112	118	123	128	133	138	143	148	153	158	163	168	174	179	184	189	194	199	204	209	215	220	225	230	235	240	245	250	255	261	266	271	276
61	100	106	111	116	122	127	132	137	143	148	153	158	164	169	174	180	185	190	195	201	206	211	217	222	227	232	238	243	248	254	259	264	269	275	280	285
62	104	109	115	120	126	131	136	142	147	153	158	164	169	175	180	186	191	196	202	207	213	218	224	229	235	240	246	251	256	262	267	273	278	284	289	295
63	107	113	118	124	130	135	141	146	152	157	163	169	175	180	186	191	197	203	208	214	220	225	231	237	242	248	254	259	265	270	278	282	287	293	299	304
64	110	116	122	128	134	140	145	151	156	162	168	174	180	186	192	197	204	209	215	221	227	232	238	244	250	256	262	267	273	279	285	291	296	302	308	314
65	114	120	126	132	138	144	150	156	162	168	174	180	186	192	198	204	210	216	222	228	234	240	246	252	258	264	270	276	282	288	294	300	306	312	318	324
66	118	124	130	136	142	148	155	161	167	173	179	186	192	198	204	210	216	223	229	235	241	247	253	260	266	272	278	284	291	297	303	309	315	322	328	334
67	121	127	134	140	146	153	159	166	172	178	185	191	198	204	211	217	223	230	236	242	249	255	261	268	274	280	287	293	299	306	312	319	325	331	338	344
68	125	131	138	144	151	158	164	171	177	184	190	197	203	210	216	223	230	236	243	249	256	262	269	276	282	289	295	302	308	315	322	328	335	341	348	354
69	128	135	142	149	155	162	169	176	182	189	196	203	209	216	223	230	236	243	250	257	263	270	277	284	291	297	304	311	318	324	331	338	345	351	358	365
70	132	139	146	153	160	167	174	181	188	195	202	209	216	222	229	236	243	250	257	264	271	278	285	292	299	306	313	320	327	334	341	348	355	362	369	376
71	136	143	150	157	165	172	179	186	193	200	208	215	222	229	236	243	250	257	265	272	279	286	293	301	308	315	322	329	336	343	351	358	365	372	379	386
72	140	147	154	162	169	177	184	191	199	206	213	221	228	235	242	250	258	265	272	279	287	294	302	309	316	324	331	338	346	353	361	368	375	383	390	397
73	144	151	159	166	174	182	189	197	204	212	219	227	235	242	250	257	265	272	280	288	295	302	310	318	325	333	340	348	355	363	371	378	386	393	401	408
74	148	155	163	171	179	186	194	202	210	218	225	233	241	249	256	264	272	280	287	295	303	311	319	326	334	342	350	358	365	373	381	389	396	404	412	420
75	152	160	168	176	184	192	200	208	216	224	232	240	248	256	264	272	279	287	295	303	311	319	327	335	343	351	359	367	375	383	391	399	407	415	423	431
76	156	164	172	180	189	197	205	213	221	230	238	246	254	263	271	279	287	295	304	312	320	328	336	344	353	361	369	377	385	394	402	410	418	426	435	443

in weight can make a drastic difference in a woman's ability to conceive, so Susie may begin to see improvements in her fertility after losing as little as 17 pounds!

If you need to lose weight in order to improve your odds of conception, the most important thing is to make sure the diet plan you use is supportive of fertility. For this reason we suggest that you read on about the kinds of foods and eating habits that promote fertility and make sure that any diet you use takes these tenets into consideration.

STEP 2. ESSENTIAL NUTRIENTS FOR FERTILITY: THE MACRO AND THE MICRO

What sets a fertility diet apart is that the food choices we make are specific to our goal of becoming pregnant. When nutritionists talk about foods, they often break them into groups called macronutrients. Macronutrients are the source of calories that our bodies use for energy as well as the basic building blocks of food.

There are three major macronutrients: carbohydrate, fat, and protein. The most calorie-dense macronutrient is fat. Gram for gram, fat provides more than double the calories of carbohydrate or protein. One gram of fat provides 9 calories, whereas carbohydrate and protein each provide 4 calories per gram. Micronutrients, more commonly known as vitamins and minerals, are essential to good physiological function, but are required in much smaller amounts than macronutrients. Nutritionists stress that micronutrients are best obtained through the diet, since human beings evolved eating food rather than dietary supplements. In addition, food scientists are constantly discovering new compounds in foods that have health benefits. To forego a fresh, balanced diet rich in fruits and vegetables in exchange for supplement tablets is short-sighted. The trick to eating a fertility-friendly diet is to maximize the micronutrient content of the calories we consume—in other words to get as many vitamins and minerals per calorie as we can. Nutritionists call this concept nutrient density, or "bang for the calorie buck."

Fertility-Smart Carbohydrates

A fully fertile diet is filled with vegetables, fruit, and whole grains. For the most part, these are carbohydrate-containing foods. Carbohydrates are the sugars, fibers, and starches that our body converts to glucose, our body's primary source of energy. Carbohydrates can be divided into two categories, simple and complex.

Simple carbohydrates are sugars that are absorbed quickly by the body and have low nutrient density (any kind of sugar, honey, molasses, candy), high fructose corn syrup (soft drinks, processed cookies and sweets, ketchup), highly refined grains like white flour and rice, fruit sugars, and milk sugars (lactose). Simple carbs should be limited.

Complex carbohydrates contain fiber and are absorbed more slowly by the body. These are the foods that we emphasize in the fertility diet. Complex carbohydrates include whole grains, whole-grain breads, beans and lentils, fruit (the whole thing, not juice or "natural sweeteners" like fruit sugars), as well as starchy vegetables such as squash, potatoes, sweet potatoes, etc.

Whole grains are nutrient-dense. They are an important source of the B vitamins that help to support our reproductive hormone function. In addition to whole grains, other complex carbohydrates such as beans and lentils can help to regulate blood sugar. Choose whole-grain foods to get the nutritional benefits from the entire grain—the bran, the germ, and the endosperm. Whole grains add fiber to the diet in addition to carbohydrates, vitamins, and minerals.

Fiber is a non-caloric complex carbohydrate found in coarse, indigestible plant matter also known as "roughage." Fiber is found in some fruits, most vegetables, and whole-grain foods. There are actually two kinds of fiber that act in very different ways in the body. Neither enters the bloodstream but rather work their magic in the colon.

Soluble fiber dissolves in water and forms a gel which helps to slow the emptying of food from the stomach and thus regulates blood sugar. It is found in foods such as oats, oat bran, barley, rye, beans, peas, and other legumes, vegetables and fresh fruits like apples and pears. Soluble fiber also binds with fatty acids and draws them out of our body. Soluble fibers have been shown to reduce total cholesterol and LDL (bad) cholesterol.

Insoluble fiber does not dissolve in water and includes wheat bran, whole-grain cereals, skins of dried beans, peas, potatoes, fruits, nuts, seeds, cauliflower, and green beans. Insoluble fiber helps regulate bowel function. Insoluble fiber helps to decrease transit time of food in the large intestine, thus speeding the elimination of toxins from the body. Both kinds of fiber increase the satiety value of food, making us feel fuller faster and curbing hunger, which is a great thing if you're watching your calories.

The recommended daily intake of fiber is 25 grams. While fiber is important for fertility, studies done in breast cancer survivors have shown that major increases in fiber (> 29 g) caused a significant decrease in serum bio-available estrogen. This is a good thing for breast cancer, and for overweight women who are trying to conceive, both of whom benefit from a reduction of circulating estrogen. However, for normal-weight women, excessive fiber intake (> 25 g) may adversely affect hormone levels. Many of the best vegetables for fertility (broccoli, cauliflower, cooking greens, squashes) consist of little more than fiber, vitamins, and minerals. The wonderful thing about these foods is that they are quite nutrient-dense and can provide enormous nutritional value without excess calories.

A big question that many women have regarding carbohydrates when they are trying to conceive is how much dietary carbohydrate is optimal for fertility. There is an emerging body of science that suggests that lower carbohydrate diets may improve blood sugar regulation and ovarian hormonal levels in women with Polycystic Ovarian Syndrome.

In these studies, carbohydrate content of the lower carb diets was about 40–45 percent of calories. While these studies are interesting and encouraging, it is important to stress that *low carbohydrate does not mean low vegetable, fruit, and whole-grain diets*. The kinds of carbohydrates you choose may be as important as the amount of carbohydrate you eat. If you are eating a diet rich in vegetables and whole grains and avoiding processed grains and sugar, you are on the right track for optimal fertility.

Fertile Woman: Know Thy Fats

As a macronutrient, fat has been much maligned in recent years. In the late eighties and early nineties, very low-fat diets (many recommending a fat intake as low as 10 percent of total calories) became all the rage and the marketplace flooded with fat-free versions of fat-containing foods. Unfortunately, these low-fat products were high in sugar and contributed to our national trend towards obesity and Type 2 Diabetes. As often happens, this low-fat fad was followed by a high-fat craze that encouraged dieters to eat bacon, steaks, and lobster dipped in butter instead of eating rice cakes. Now the pendulum has swung back to center with the realization that fat is an important part of our diet because it provides food with flavor and satiety value, and new research shows that certain kinds of fats may actually promote good health. Our intake of fat should be approached moderately and intelligently, however. Whatever the health benefits of fats, they do remain the most calorie-dense macronutrient. With such a high "calorie cost" it is important that we consume the right *kinds* of fat and fully understand the differences in fats and fatty acids.

Fats are either *saturated, unsaturated,* or *transaturated* and different fats contain different fatty acids. *Saturated fats* are solid at room temperature and include butter, lard, and white fat (marbling) on meat, and full-fat dairy products. Coconut and palm kernel oil are also high in saturated fat and should be considered as solid fats. Diets high in saturated fats are implicated in heart disease and some cancers and for optimal fertility we aim to limit our intake of saturated fat. *Unsaturated fats* are liquid at room temperature and sources include oils, nuts, and avocadoes. They are further broken down into monounsaturated and polyunsaturated fats. Mono- and polyunsaturated fats have received attention in recent years for their potential health benefits.

Monounsaturated fats are liquid at room temperature but start to become solid in the refrigerator. Examples include avocado, canola and olive oil, olives, nuts (almonds and cashews), peanuts, peanut butter, sesame seeds, and tahini, or sesame paste. *Polyunsaturated fats* are liquid at room temperature and in the refrigerator. Examples include walnut, corn, sesame, safflower, and soybean oil, pumpkin and sunflower seeds, and fish oils. There are two essential polyunsaturated fatty acids, omega-6 (linoleic) and omega-3 (linolenic), that we obtain through dietary unsaturated fats. Ideally, our intake of omega-6 fats should be no more than 4–5 times our intake of omega-3s. Unfortunately, a typical American diet is providing about 14–15 times more omega-6 fats which can lead to inflammation and other negative consequences.

Trans fats are produced when liquid fats such as oils are converted by chemical means into semi-soft solids during a process called hydrogenation. An example of this is stick margarine in addition to French fries, donuts, cookies, crackers, and commercial baked goods. Unfortunately, increasing clinical evidence shows that the human body is ill-equipped to metabolize this new-fangled fat. High intake of trans fats has been linked with heart disease cancer and now ovulatory infertility as evidenced by findings from the Nurses Health Study. Experts theorize that our high consumption of trans fats (they're everywhere!) creates an environment where trans fats compete with other dietary fats for our body's crucial fat-metabolizing enzymes and that trans fats are becoming integrated into our body's fatty components such as cell membranes and our fat cells. It's even possible that trans fats contribute to insulin resistance. Insulin receptors perch in the lipid bi-layer that surrounds all of our cells. If trans fats are infiltrating this important barrier, cells may become less efficient in their ability to manage blood sugar. For this reason "trans free" products are now being produced and trans fats are an absolute "no" when you're trying to conceive.

Our "fat strategy" for fertility is to choose foods rich in mono- and polyunsaturated fats, particularly the omega-3 fats that are deficient in the typical American diet, to limit intake of saturated fat, and to *dramatically* decrease—read eliminate!—intake of trans fat. Experiment with different oils and nuts to increase your intake of healthy fats. Many of us have shied away from nuts because of their high calorie and fat content. But nuts are high in omega-3 essential fatty acids as well as other vitamins and minerals. If it's just too hard to control your nut intake, try adding nut butters to hot cereal or your morning toast. The fat in nuts will also help to slow down the transit of food from stomach to intestines, increasing the satiety value of your meal, as well as help to control the after-meal rise in blood sugar.

Good Protein Choices for Conception

Dietary protein is the nutrient which is essential for the growth and repair of tissues and is critical for optimal fertility. While protein is found in many animal products such as red meat, pork, poultry, fish, eggs, and dairy products (milk, yogurt, and cheese), and in plant foods including beans, nuts, seeds, and soy products, not all protein sources are created equal when it comes to fertility.

Surprisingly, even though we embrace yoga philosophy, we do not endorse vegetarianism when a woman is trying to conceive (please see Our Beef with Vegetarianism Box on p. 96). The healing sciences of Ayurveda and OM that inform much of our understanding of what's good and what's not good for fertility both suggest that it is appropriate to supplement the diet with animal protein when the body is in metabolic need. At PDtM we include the process of trying to conceive in this category of metabolic need. The wisdom of these teachings appears to be born out by clinical studies that have demonstrated greater incidence of menstrual irregularity in vegetarian women when compared to non-vegetarian women. For these reasons, our guiding principles for fertility-friendly protein are to eat varied sources of protein including beans, poultry, eggs, lean meats, and non-fatty fish. Of course any animal products should be low in saturated fat and come from free-range, pasture-fed animals. Other forms of dietary protein, including dairy and soy, will be discussed later in the chapter.

Our Beef with Vegetarianism

Vegetarianism has gained popularity in recent years, ignited, perhaps, by two distinct influences on our culture. The first is Dr. Dean Ornish, the famous cardiologist and author of five best-selling books who was the first to claim that heart disease and clogged arteries can be controlled and even cleared through diet, exercise and stress management techniques. Through his own research findings and personal experience, Dr. Ornish concludes that eating a vegetarian diet with only 10 percent of the total daily calories from fat is the first step necessary to leading a happy and healthier life.

The second influence is the increasing number of people who are becoming more and more educated on the deplorable living conditions and inhumane treatment experienced by so many animals across the globe. It is no secret that animals today are being fed more toxic food laced with pesticides, are living in unsanitary conditions, and are being injected with growth hormones and antibiotics which ultimately end up being ingested by humans. Diseases such as mad cow and bird flu also have us rightfully concerned over the safety of eating animal flesh.

Yoga Philosophy and Vegetarianism

From the perspective of yoga philosophy, the reason for vegetarianism is stated in the Yoga Sutras, an ancient text dating back to the first century BCE. In this sacred scripture, author Patanjali offers a series of practices that help guide individuals to ultimate bliss and liberation from earthly suffering. One of these practices is Ahimsa which is a Sanskrit word that translates to mean "non-violence." Non-violence is an undertaking to live your life without causing harm or injury to another living thing in thought, word, or action. Not only should you avoid causing harm to others, you should do what you can to bring happiness into their lives. This is why so many yogis are vegetarians. They believe that the killing of animals for food is a form of violence to both society and the earth.

Unfortunately, too many people practice the letter of the law but miss the spirit of the law. Practicing ahimsa by avoiding meat but then cussing out your co-worker or speaking negatively about a friend is still a form of violence. You can give up filet mignon, but if you feel like you want to strangle your doctor with his stethoscope, you still have lots of work to do. This is one of our "beefs with vegetarianism." Don't be a hypocrite. If you don't eat chickens but you experience road rage once a week and are impatient with the grocery clerk, you really aren't contributing much to saving the world or making society a more peaceful place. Start out small while still doing what you can to make the Earth a better place to live. Practice patience, love, compassion, and kindness to all living creatures you come into contact with. Learn to forgive your enemies and yourself. Once you have mastered that you can stop eating the animals.

Eating Meat Responsibly

Putting yoga philosophy aside for a moment, it is interesting to note that some of the most devout monks in the Himalayas are yak eaters. If man was meant to eat only fruits and vegetables, why do we not have teeth like a rabbit? Why, in nature, is there a food chain? Should a cheetah practice vegetarianism to truly be enlightened? Is all meat bad meat?

If you are bothered, as we are, by the horrific living conditions and treatment of animals, research local vendors in your area that carry organic, free-range, hormone-free, grain-fed meats. Even your eggs and milk should be hormone- and antibiotic-free. Make a commitment to yourself and to your environment to spend a little extra time and money each week in order to do the right thing for your body and for your brother/sister animals.

The pros and cons of vegetarianism are often debated by our students and patients at PDtM. Ultimately, the choice to give up animal protein is as individual as how you like your steak done. If you do decide to continue eating meat don't forget to say a prayer of gratitude before you consume it. When you sit down to dinner, honor the cow, the chicken, the pig, or the fish by acknowledging that it has given its life to nourish your body. Be thankful, be gracious, and never be wasteful. And when you're done, refrain from screaming at your spouse for never cleaning the dishes.

Prayer before your meal

If you are not a vegetarian (and even if you are), it's a good idea to say a prayer of thanksgiving before you begin your meal. From a yoga philosopher's point of view, when you consume an animal, you are also consuming some of the karma that goes along with it. We are sure you can understand that eating a carrot has fewer karmic ramifications than consuming a cow or pig. Offering a prayer of thanksgiving to the animal softens some of that karma. You might try a prayer like this one:

> I thank you, the animal that has given its life so that my physical body
> might be nourished and fed. I, in turn, will try to nourish and feed others
> so that you have not died in vain but rather have contributed to the
> betterment of all humankind.

Regardless of the philosophical reasons for praying before your meal there are some practical reasons as well. Praying gives us pause in our day; an opportunity to look at and appreciate our food before we consume it. It gives us a snapshot of what we are about to put into our bodies and provides an opportunity to bring mindfulness into our meal. Express gratitude in your mealtime prayer. Even if you don't feel especially grateful for your food, find something else from the context of your day for which to be grateful and state it. When you say your prayer, whether silently or aloud, try using the hand position pictured below. This mudra or hand gesture is called the Shanti Mudra, or gesture of blessing. It is performed by taking the middle finger (Saturn finger) and placing it on top of the first finger (Jupiter finger). You then touch these fingers to your plate or anything else that you wish to bless. By touching your plate before your meal, you are sending positive vibrations into the food. As you touch the plate say, "Om, shanti, shanti, shanti." Shanti is the Sanskrit word for peace. If we explore this mudra a bit further we see that, in yoga, the thumb represents God or the universe. By placing your thumb on the plate you are expressing gratitude to God or acknowledging that all of this comes from that (the Divine). The first finger is then placed on the plate which represents the planet Jupiter. Jupiter is known as the planet of abundance. May you continue to have abundance of food, shelter and all things necessary for life. The middle finger is the Saturn finger. This planet is known to be the worker and the grounding energy. It reminds us that although abundance flows, it should never be taken for granted because all life can and will be difficult or challenging. Using this hand gesture on your plate before you eat is a prayer unto itself.

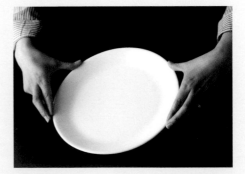

Meat and Fish

Grass-fed beef has a healthier profile of omega fatty acids than corn-fed beef. In comparison to corn-fed beef, which has an omega 6:3 ratio of more than 20:1, grass-fed beef has a ratio of 0.16:1, a ratio similar to fish. In addition, cattle raised in this way have not been fed or injected with added hormones. Other meats such as bison, pork, and ostrich can be consumed in moderation but always look for grass-fed varieties.

By USDA definition, free-range poultry should have access to the outdoors during their lives. There is no definition for free-range eggs, and unscrupulous farmers may attach this name to chickens which simply have a window in their cage or coop. Unlike grass-fed beef, free-range chickens are more likely to have eaten a great deal of grain—because many cage-free birds are allowed to roam in a fenced enclosure that, while certainly an improvement over tiny cages, is still a manner of mass production. Where possible, look for pastured chickens, which are put to pasture and graze on grass, and the bugs who eat grass, as well as some grain feed.

Navigating the Fish Counter

The Catch-22 of the fish counter is that fish is a wonderful source of protein that contains omega-3 fatty acids, which we've learned are great for fertility as well as pregnancy. However, like all foods, fish carry risks of contamination by pesticides, mercury, and PCBs. The amount of mercury in fish that is considered "safe" by the FDA is controversial and double that accepted as safe by the Environment Protection Agency and Canada.

Fish for Fertility

These omega-3 rich fish can be safely consumed twice a week:

- *Salmon (all varieties except from the Great Lakes, or farm-raised)*
- *Farmed trout*
- *Sardines*
- *Pilchard*
- *Herring*

These fish are lower in omega-3s but are lower in contaminants and safely consumed twice a week:
- *Flounder and sole*
- *Farm-raised catfish, striped bass, tilapia*
- *Cod*
- *Haddock*
- *Mahi mahi*
- *Perch*
- *Crab, shrimp, scallops, clams, oysters, mussels, crayfish*

(Source: Nettleton, 2002)

Not all fish is created equal, however. Because of its age, size, and predatory nature (eating little fish), tuna is under the microscope for contamination. Both canned and fresh tuna are at risk and should be limited in the fertility diet. Other fish to be avoided are large sport fish such as swordfish, shark, king mackerel, and tile fish (also called golden bass or golden snapper). For fertility, a bigger fish definitely isn't better.

STEP 3: GOOD BLOOD SUGAR CONTROL

As mentioned at the beginning of this chapter, our ovaries are quite sensitive to insulin, the hormone that regulates blood sugar. When levels of this hormone become higher than normal, insulin can "invade" hormone receptors on the ovaries that are designed for reproductive hormones and disrupt communication in the HPO (hypothalamic-pituitary-ovarian axis). In addition, high levels of insulin can cause the cells in the ovarian tissues to over-produce androgens, such as testosterone. Effects such as these disrupt the delicate balance of the reproductive system and can make it harder for a woman to conceive.

To ensure that our body is producing insulin in a judicious manner—only when needed and at the lowest necessary level to get the job done—we want to avoid "peaks and valleys" in our blood sugar. Too often our eating habits don't support good blood sugar regulation, as we can see in this day-in-the-life of fertility patient, Susie Q:

Susie is a sugar junkie. She just loves sweets, from her Starbuck's maple scone in the morning to the chocolate chip cookie she nibbles after dinner. Her afternoon snack of a granola bar is low-fat, but chock full of sugar. No matter how much she tries, she can't stop the sugar cravings. Her weight is normal, but it seems she's always ravenous. Susie knows she shouldn't be eating all this sugar, but what she may not realize is that her eating habits may also be creating a situation that is bad not only for her overall health but for her fertility as well. Let's take a closer look at what's happening as Susie goes through her day.

Susie is the first to admit she eats too many sweets, but she feels she can't help it. This is because each sugary meal or snack quickly causes her blood sugar to rise to a high level. In response, the pancreas secretes insulin, actually "overshooting" the level necessary to return blood sugar to its normal level, and blood sugar levels drop too low. This in turn stimulates a craving for more sugar, creating a vicious cycle that repeatedly exposes the ovaries to high levels of insulin, with the risk of eventually causing insulin resistance, a condition where our cells lose the ability to respond to insulin, and potentially resulting in impaired reproductive function.

Tips for Steady Blood Sugar

There are diet strategies we can use to keep our blood sugar under control and to avoid the roller-coaster ride that perpetuates sugar cravings:

- Eat regular meals and snacks, avoid long periods of fasting.
- Cut back on sugary treats and drinks.
- Foods high in soluble fiber (whole grains, dried beans and peas, oat bran, barley, nuts, fruits—apples, oranges, pears—and vegetables) help to control blood sugar.
- Consume some healthy fat or lean protein along with carbohydrates.
  This will help slow the digestion and assimilation of sugars into the blood stream. Try a tablespoon of peanut or almond butter on some wheat toast, or have some guacamole with whole wheat pita chips instead of a sugary granola bar.

STEP 4: FERTILITY GO FOODS AND NO FOODS

Go Big "O": The Importance of Organic

The fertility diet is a hormone-free diet. This is because hormones or hormone-like chemicals consumed in our diet or through our environment can disrupt the function of our reproductive system. Some hormone intake through the diet is inevitable and even natural, but with the increasing amounts of hormone-like substances in our diet and environment, it is difficult to know where the "tipping point" lies.

Eating organic meat, poultry, eggs, and dairy products is a good way to start minimizing your consumption of hormones and additives. These products come from animals which are raised without antibiotics or growth hormones. Organic vegetables and grains are grown without application of pesticides, synthetic fertilizers or sewage sludge, bioengineering, or ionizing radiation. As of 2002, producers of foods labeled organic, as well as processors of such foods, must have been inspected and cleared by an independent, government-approved certifier. Look for the USDA Organic seal for a product that is guaranteed to be at least 95 percent organic. In the UK look for the Soil Association's logo for a similar guarantee.

Organic food has also been grown and produced with a commitment to renewable resources and the conservation of soil and water to enhance environmental quality for future generations. You may also want to check into the availability of organic co-op farms or crop-shares in your area. These smaller, wholly organic, and farmer-owned outfits are often an economical and earth-friendly route to eating organic.

TABLE 3.2 PESTICIDE RESIDUES IN FRUIT

HIGHEST PESTICIDE RESIDUE

Fruit/vegetable	Major nutrient	Nutritional "match" with lower pesticide residues
Strawberries	Vitamin C	Blackberries, raspberries, blueberries, kiwi, orange, cantaloupe
Bell peppers		
Green	Vitamin C	Green peas, broccoli, romaine lettuce
Red	Vitamin C, Vitamin A	Carrots, broccoli, Brussels sprouts, tomatoes, asparagus, romaine lettuce
Cherries (US)	Vitamin C	Grapefruit, blueberries, raspberries, cantaloupe, oranges
Peaches	Vitamin C, Vitamin A	Nectarines, canned peaches, cantaloupe (US), tangerine, grapefruit, watermelon
Cantaloupe (Mexico)	Vitamin C, Vitamin A, Potassium	Watermelon, cantaloupe (US)
Celery	Carotenoids	Carrots, broccoli, radishes, romaine lettuce
Apples	Vitamin C, Vitamin A, Potassium	Oranges, nectarines, bananas, kiwis, watermelon
Apricots	Vitamin C, Vitamin A, Potassium	Nectarines, cantaloupe (US), watermelon, tangerines, grapefruit
Green beans	Carotenoids	Green peas, broccoli, cauliflower, brussels sprouts, asparagus
Grapes (Chile)	Vitamin C, Potassium	Grapes (US), in season
Cucumbers	Vitamin A, Potassium	Carrots, romaine lettuce, broccoli, radishes
Pears	Vitamin A, Vitamin C, Folic Acid	Canned pears, canned peaches, oranges, nectarines
Winter squash (US)	Vitamin A, Vitamin C, Folic Acid, Potassium	Winter squash (Honduras, Mexico), sweet potatoes (US)
Potatoes (US)	Vitamin C, Folic Acid	Sweet potatoes (US), carrots, winter squash (Honduras, Mexico)

LOWEST PESTICIDE RESIDUE

Avocados	Grapes (US)
Corn	Bananas
Onions	Plums
Sweet potatoes	Green onions
Cauliflower	Watermelon
Brussels sprouts	Broccoli

Pesticides and Toxins

What is known about the harmful effects of pesticides is based on studies that focused not on whether long-term, low-dose exposures to these chemicals are safe, but rather from high-dose studies that were designed to ferret out gross toxic effects. The main concern for fertility is whether consuming these chemicals steadily and at low concentrations can be harmful. Absence of knowledge is *not* proof of safety. By definition, pesticides are designed to be toxic and our goal for optimal fertility is to reduce toxicity.

Pesticides and artificial growth hormones have been shown to cause hormone disruption in both women and men. They bind to hormone receptor cells and either mimic or block hormone action, with the potential to promote estrogen-related cancers, infertility, and endometriosis. A recent study examined 49 commonly used pesticides and found 15 that interacted with estrogen receptors. The most worrisome of these chemicals are called xeno-estrogens and xeno-androgens. (*Lemaire, 2006*)

Table 3.2 shows which fruits and vegetables have the highest pesticide residues and suggests nutritional twins—other items you can eat which may have similar vitamins and minerals but lower pesticide residues. The table is compiled from data from studies by Consumers Union, the publishers of *Consumer Report,* and the Environmental Working Group, using data from the US Food and Drug Administration. The Consumers Union found that pesticide residue is concentrated in a relatively small number of fruit and vegetables, often from differing geographical regions.

The Soy Dilemma

So what about soy, the godsend of vegetarians everywhere? In addition to being a convenient and highly bio-available source of vegetable protein, soy has lately enjoyed the reputation of being a sort of "miracle food." Promising studies done on heart disease and breast cancer in the 1990s showed potential health benefits to eating foods containing soy protein. Epidemiologists studying the lower rates of breast cancer in Asian women suggested this might be a function of diet; in particular, intake of soy foods like tofu and miso. Researchers hypothesized that much of the health benefits of soy come from substances that have a chemical structure similar to estrogen and are called isoflavones. Two isoflavones in particular, genistein and diadzein, are credited with a strong estrogenic effect. Isoflavones are postulated to exert an effect in the body similar to the cancer-prevention drug tamoxifen by blocking our cells' estrogen receptors. Obviously, while this may be great for preventing breast cancer, it's not so good for fertility.

There is a body of clinical research that suggests that soy may be detrimental to fertility in both males and females. In addition, a limited number of feeding studies in human females have shown soy diets to lower ovarian hormone levels. Most of these studies were designed

Fertility-Friendly Food Choices

Apart from making the best possible choices and considering alternatives where available, here are some strategies you can use to make your fruits and vegetables more fertility-friendly and cut your toxin intake substantially:

- *Buy organic, local, and in-season.*
- *Wash both organic and non-organic vegetables and fruit with a produce wash. You can buy one at your local grocery store or make your own using 1 gallon of water and 1 teaspoon environmentally safe dishwashing detergent (sold in health food stores). Grapes, berries, green beans, and leafy greens should be swirled for 5-10 seconds and then rinsed in clear water. Other fruits and vegetables can be scrubbed with a soft brush for 5–10 seconds and then rinsed.*
- *Peel fruits and vegetables with higher pesticide risk (some chemicals can penetrate skin).*
- *Surprisingly, frozen non-organic vegetables are less of a pesticide risk than fresh non-organic vegetables. The power washing process prior to freezing is quite thorough and removes a fair amount of chemicals.*
- *Grow your own.*

to tease out soy's potential role in the prevention of breast cancer. They examined such outcome variables as cycle length and reproductive hormone levels rather than time to conception or fertility rates. (*Cassidy, 1994; Lulu, 1996; 2001*)

The problem is, there are no studies that actually examine the impact of soy on rates of infertility or pregnancy outcomes in humans. Women in Asian countries, where soy has been consumed as part of the traditional diet for generations, do not have higher rates of infertility than here in the States. Nevertheless, the way that soy has entered the American diet scene is different from ways in which it is consumed in Asian countries. In this country we eat a lot of soy protein in the form of veggie burgers, meat-alternative products, TVP (textured vegetable protein), energy bars, and soy milk. This is quite different from the way soy is consumed in countries where it is part of the traditional eating patterns.

Until there is more conclusive clinical evidence about soy's impact on fertility, we recommend limiting soy intake to one serving per day. Soy is now added to so many foods (breads, breakfast cereals, prepared meals, energy bars, etc.) that we feel that even women who choose to follow this advice to limit their soy intake to a few servings a week run little danger of a soy "deficiency," if such a thing exists. For vegetarians and vegans, this guideline may make finding adequate protein sources a challenge. Our heart-felt advice to women who are currently vegetarian is to consider suspending their vegetarian diet while they're trying to conceive (see Our Beef with Vegetarianism, p. 96). If this is not acceptable, ovo-lacto vegetarians can consider supplementing their diets with protein powders and shakes based on organic whey protein. Vegans may wish to experiment with other non-dairy/non-soy protein sources such as rice protein or quinoa. How's that for the next great Starbuck's drink? "I'll have a vente vegan no-soy extra-high-protein shake, please!"

Dairy

In accordance with the same hormone-free philosophy with which we approach organics and soy, we recommend limiting dairy consumption to a few servings a week. The milk we drink today contains not only added growth hormones; it also contains the naturally present reproductive hormones of the female cow at higher levels than in years past.

A recent review of clinical evidence linking consumption of cow's milk with higher incidence of hormone-related cancers led researchers to point a finger towards the modern agri-business practice of milking pregnant cows late into the gestational period. According to this review, milk from a pregnant cow can contain up to 33 percent more estrogen than milk from a cow that is not pregnant. (*Ganmaa, 2005*) Another group of researchers compared estrogen levels of raw and processed milk from non-pregnant and pregnant cows and found the lowest levels of estrogens in raw milk from non-pregnant cows. The highest levels came from the milk of pregnant cows. The level of estrogen in processed milk, which generally contains a blend of milk from pregnant and non-pregnant cows, was on par with raw milk from cows in the first and second trimester of pregnancy. The researchers concluded the daily intake of estrogen from milk is "dramatically more than currently recognized." (*Malekinejad, 2006*) Data for the National Nurses Study 2 also found that the consumption of low-fat dairy was linked to ovulatory infertility. (*Chavarro, 2007*)

Because the jury is still out on this topic, we recommend limiting the amount of dairy consumed as part of your fertility diet to one 8 oz serving per day. If you just love a glass of milk with dinner, let it be a treat and choose the (mostly) hormone-free organic kind.

Caffeine

Getting off caffeine can be a challenge but we recommend that women lose their dependence on this stimulant when they're trying to conceive. While some sources suggest that a caffeine intake of < 300 mg per day (about the amount in two or three cups of coffee) appears not to affect a woman's fertility, other studies have found that women who consume more than 300 mg of caffeine per day took longer to conceive.

Despite contradictory data, the Fully Fertile view of caffeine is that it is not a good choice when you're trying to conceive. Artificial stimulants create imbalance in our body's systems. Drinking caffeinated beverages can also make it harder for us to relax and may exacerbate poor sleeping habits as well as camouflage the effects of sleep deprivation. Furthermore, you'll have to give it up anyway once you're pregnant. And while the goose is giving up her daily cup, the gander better not laugh too hard. Research indicates that men who consume more than three cups of coffee per day had increased DNA damage in their sperm.

There are many different strategies for getting off caffeine, but one that we like is to first make the transition from coffee to green tea, which is filled with antioxidants and has lower caffeine content than coffee. Then, gradually, begin to alternate your cups of green tea with herbal teas, until the switch to herbal tea is complete.

Alcohol

Between you, us, and the cat, it's okay to enjoy a glass of wine once in a while when you're trying to conceive. But we do mean once in a while, and will be even more specific when we recommend that you keep your intake of alcoholic beverages to one to two per week. Clinical research suggests that alcohol intake negatively impacts IVF success, is associated with a longer time to conception and is associated with increased miscarriage risk. For men, chronic alcohol consumption negatively impacts sperm quality and binge drinking, particularly in men, can have a disastrous impact on fertility by causing acute drops in sperm count.

Smoking

Of course smoking is an absolute fertility "no!" for both women and men. Read more about Stop Smoking Strategies on p. 173.

STEP 5: SUPPLEMENTS FOR FERTILITY

As we mentioned before, vitamins and minerals are best obtained through the diet, since human beings evolved eating food rather than dietary supplements. In addition, since most micronutrients act in concert with other compounds found in foods, any nutrient supplementation should be mindful of the fact that vitamins and minerals are part of a complex metabolic system. That said, there are several micronutrients that are important for optimal reproductive function in women and in men. In addition, certain lifestyle factors like oral contraceptive use can put women at risk of having impaired micronutrient status and in some cases supplementation may be merited. There are four supplements that we commonly recommend for our patients: a good-quality prenatal vitamin, an antioxidant formula for men, fish oil, and a probiotic.

What about Wheat?

Should you avoid wheat when you're trying to conceive? It's a question we're often asked at PDtM. Much of the flap around wheat and infertility stems from a connection between celiac disease, a condition in which an individual cannot tolerate gluten (a protein found naturally in wheat and used as an additive in many foods) and infertility in both sexes. It is estimated that 48 percent of women with undiagnosed infertility suffer from celiac disease; and men with celiac disease have a higher risk of sub-fertility and impotence.

Celiac Disease

While the mechanism by which celiac disease impairs fertility is not fully understood, scientists have made educated guesses as to the link. Celiac disease is auto-immune in nature. If an individual is genetically predisposed to celiac disease, dietary intake of gluten (a protein found in many grains) causes a two-fold attack in the small intestine. Antibodies first attack the gluten protein and this attack triggers an autoimmune response in which antibodies attack the endomysium, a smooth muscle component in the small intestine, and damage the tiny, fingerlike protrusions on the wall of the small intestine that serve to absorb nutrients from food called villi. This leads to the most likely link between celiac disease and infertility—the malabsorption of nutrients, in particular iron and folic acid. Iron deficiency can lead to anemia (a condition that is common in persons with celiac disease). Iron deficiency has recently been implicated in ovulatory infertility and iron-containing proteins play an important role in the release and transport of the ovum at the time of ovulation.

There are two ways of testing for celiac disease. The first, through a blood test, is used in cases where celiac disease is less likely (no family history). The second and more invasive test, small intestine biopsy, is used in cases where family history of the disease is present and the likelihood of disease is higher. Celiac disease is most often successfully treated with a gluten-free diet. In the rare cases that the disease does not respond, steroid medications are used. While widespread testing for celiac disease is not yet recommended in the medical fertility field, if you or your partner manifest symptoms of Irritable Bowel Syndrome (IBS), or have a close relative who has been diagnosed with celiac disease, you may want to speak to your physician about being tested for gluten intolerance. Clinical data suggests that infertile women with celiac disease can be successfully treated with a gluten-free diet.

The elimination of wheat from the diet can be a challenging proposition. For this reason we don't recommend that women go "wheat free" without good reason. We do, however, recommend that women make a variety of grain choices—rice, millet, barley, quinoa—in their overall dietary intake.

Prenatal Vitamins for Women

A good prenatal vitamin is essential for all women who are trying to conceive, but is especially critical for women who are coming off oral contraceptives. Clinical data suggests that women who are taking oral contraceptives have lower serum levels of several nutrients that are important for fertility, including Vitamins B-6, B-2, folate, and Vitamin C. The levels of these vitamins in women on birth control pills are not at the level of deficiency, but researchers have hypothesized that the compromised nutrient status may play a role in the heart disease risk, depression symptoms, and fatigue reported by some women on the Pill. In addition to providing adequate intake of iron, calcium, and antioxidant vitamins, your prenatal vitamin will also bolster levels of folate, an essential B vitamin for pregnancy and, if you're depleted in the Bs as a result of taking the Pill, your vitamins should bring you back to a more optimal, and potentiallly more fertile, nutritional status.

Antioxidant Formula for Men

Antioxidants are substances found in food that help to counteract the negative effects of *free radicals*, the harmful by-products of our body processes that use oxygen. Oxidation is a natural part of many biochemical reactions in our body, including cellular respiration (the use of oxygen in our cells to make energy), metabolism, and inflammation. Our body has a defense system equipped to deal with free radicals—an arsenal that includes antioxidant vitamins, minerals, and enzymes. However, exogenous free radicals (those that come from sources outside our own bodies) include pollution, sunlight, alcohol, smoking, strenuous exercise, and X-rays. The picture becomes clearer as we recognize that oxidative damage is the reason that a car bumper rusts, a bottle of oil left too long on the pantry shelf turns bad or a peeled apple turns brown. As our environment and lifestyles become more toxic, our body's internal antioxidant defenses may become overwhelmed. Cell membranes, proteins, and DNA are among the prime targets for oxidative damage. In terms of fertility, there's clinical evidence that free radicals may play a role in several pathologies associated with infertility including the inflammation related to endometriosis, polycystic ovarian syndrome (PCOS), and "male factor issues" including poor sperm mobility, motility, and morphology which can limit a man's fertility.

Oxidative stress in sperm may be implicated in infertility and miscarriage, even in cases where sperm motility/mobility/count are "normal." Antioxidant vitamins include vitamins C, A, and E. We do not recommend supplementing with individual antioxidant vitamins since some of these substances can be dangerous in high dosages. Most prenatal vitamins include appropriate levels of antioxidants for a woman who is trying to conceive. We recommend that men take a specially formulated fertility supplement such as Conception XR that has been specifically designed for male fertility.

Omega-3 Fatty Acid Supplement

We recommend supplementing Omega-3 fatty acids at a dosage of 600-800 mg of DHA/EPA blend. Fatty fish like tuna, salmon, shark, and mackerel are the major food sources of Omega-3 FA. Unfortunately, it is widely recommended that women who are trying to conceive limit their intake of fatty fish in order to avoid PCBs and mercury. Omega-3 fatty acids have been proven beneficial to the development of the fetal nervous system and are now being added to prenatal vitamin blends as a matter of course. Omega-3s are also precursors of hormones and important anti-inflammatory substances in the body. In-vitro studies suggest that a high Omega-3/Omega-6 ratio may suppress the survival of endometrial cells in culture and other researchers have suggested the potential benefits of Omega-3 FAs on uterine blood flow.

Probiotic Supplement

Healthy intestinal flora may support fertility by limiting yeast overgrowth, preventing vaginal yeast infections, blocking the absorption of harmful chemicals in the colon, and by improving elimination.

STEP 6: TRADITIONAL HEALING DIET

Now here's a fertility diet tip you definitely won't hear at Weight Watchers. Some of the most important qualities of PDtM's fertility diet derive from the teachings of the traditional healing sciences of OM and Ayurveda. While they differ in the details, these holistic sciences agree that a fertility diet should be:

Warming

According to both OM and Ayurveda, digestion is a warm process. By this token cooked vegetables are better for our overall health than raw. It's true that there are more nutrients in raw vegetables than in cooked, but we can actually obtain more nutrients from the slightly cooked sample. Cooking is a type of pre-digestion and makes the food more easily absorbed. Additionally, our bodies must work extra hard to warm up anything we consume in a raw or cold state. This robs valuable energy (Qi) from our digestive system and slows down the process of digestion as well as depletes our overall life-energy levels. Ditto for our penchant for ice-cold beverages. OM recommends that we drink hot beverages with our meals to facilitate digestion.

This does not mean that you can never have a salad when you're trying to conceive just don't eat one at every meal and, when you do, wash it down with some herbal tea. Many women are surprised to realize they're "addicted" to cold drinks, desserts, and cold, raw food preparation methods, and most report improved digestion with just a little "dietary warming."

Seasonal and Local

In keeping with the OM belief that we are healthier when our bodies are in tune with the cycles of nature, you should eat foods that grow in your geographical area and that are in season. Whether they are indigenous or adoptive species, plants that thrive in particular areas are there because they have established harmony with their surroundings. OM teaches that foods and people in the same geographical area have "similar energy." This may be true in the sense that plants and the people living as neighbors share the same weather, air, soil, and "roots" and therefore are connected in a larger community or ecosystem.

Prepared versus Processed

Preparing as opposed to processing foods can help us actually add Qi to our bodies through the intake of life-energy rich foods. Adding Qi to your diet can be achieved in two main ways: respecting the vitamin and nutrient content of the foods in our diet by eating minimally processed foods and learning to enjoy the act of food preparation and consumption. Making your meals a mindful and healing experience can turn a simple meal into a serious dose of Qi.

Processing versus Preparing

When traditional healers suggest that we eat food as close as possible to its natural state, they do not mean that we should snack on raw beet roots still covered in garden dirt. In fact, as discussed previously, the over-consumption of raw foods can actually stress and slow the digestive system down and drain precious prana from our body with the effort of digestion. Rather, the idea of preserving the Qi in food means learning the difference between processing and preparation. This is the difference between a baked potato and a frozen tater tot, a slice of cantaloupe and a glass of sugary fruit juice, and a homemade stir-fry and a "lean & healthy" microwave meal. Preparing preserves as much of the nutrient value of a food as possible while making a food palatable and enjoyable to eat. Processing has evolved to make food amenable to mass production, and includes chemical additives and preservatives to increase shelf-life and may involve packaging and storage issues that are harmful to both our bodies and the environment such as plastic wrappers and Styrofoam containers. According to experts, the processing of foods can cause a nutrient loss of as much as 50–80 percent. No wonder so many people in the United States are overweight and undernourished from eating calories robbed of their nutrition.

Cooking Methods and Nutrient Loss

Since we recommend that most of the food consumed as part of a fertility-friendly diet be cooked, we should take a moment to discuss cooking methods. There is a traditional piece

Nutrient-Friendly Cooking Tips

- *Steaming vegetables is less damaging to their nutrient content than boiling.*
- *Stir-fry veggies in a healthy oil.*
- *Dry heat methods like baking or roasting* *vegetables intensify flavors. With the exception of Vitamin C, roasting does not impair the nutrient status of vegetables in any significant way.*

of nutrition wisdom that when it comes to preserving the nutritional value of cooked vegetables, water and heat are the enemy. The longer a food is exposed to heat, the more its nutritional value is lost. If we're mindful of the way we cook our foods, we can keep the nutrient loss to a minimum (about 5–15 percent) and still create the favorable changes in digestibility and the conversion of nutrients into more absorbable forms that are a by-product of the cooking process.

STEP 7: WATER: GO WITH THE FLOW

Water intake is an important part of optimal health. Proper hydration ensures that metabolic processes work more effectively and water helps to detoxify the body by carrying waste out of the body in urine. To ensure you are properly hydrated, drink at least eight, 8 oz glasses of water per day, avoid caffeinated beverages, which can be dehydrating, and drink water and other beverages warm or at room temperature.

Let us repeat—water is not tea, or fruit juice, or soup broth. Water is water and should be mineral or spring water, not distilled, as the process of distillation removes important mineral content.

WEEK 3: ACTIVITY 1: KEEP A FOOD DIARY

As we discussed early on in this chapter, our overall goal for this week is to make changes to our eating patterns that are conducive to good reproductive function. Developing the best diet for your fertility will most likely require making changes in your current eating patterns (if not, good for you!). A food journal (see Table 3.3 on p. 112) is a fabulous way to a) get a baseline idea of what you're eating and see what needs to change, and b) track your progress towards a fully fertile diet. Remembering everything we eat and drink on a given day is really hard, especially when things get busy. There's food everywhere: at work, home, and on the go, so you may find that you do a fair amount of mindless snacking and grazing. By writing down what you eat, you will be aware of everything going in your mouth. Also, if you do choose to get extra help from a nutritionist, there is a wealth of information about your eating patterns or potential areas for improvement and how to correct them.

Mindful Eating

- Get a cute notebook that fits in your purse so you can keep it with you all day.
- Write down all the foods you eat for meals and snacks from the time you get up in the morning until you go to bed.
- Be sure to record portion sizes (just estimate).
- Don't forget beverages; water goes on there too!

- Very importantly, write down those sneaky, unplanned snacks. Who knows, maybe you'll be less likely to eat that cookie if you know you have to write it in the journal!
- Other tips: write down roughly the times you eat as this can also be important. You may also choose to record your exercise as well so you can keep track of how it's going.

TABLE 3.3 FULLY FERTILE NUTRITION LOG

	DAY/DATE	DAY/DATE	DAY/DATE	DAY/DATE	DAY/DATE	DAY/DATE	DAY/DATE
WAKE UP:							
MORNING MEAL:							
TIME:							
SNACK:							
TIME:							
EVENING MEAL:							
TIME:							
WATER (OUNCES):							
OTHER:							
ACTIVITY/ EXERCISE:							
WHAT KIND:							
HOW LONG:							
SLEEP TIME							

In the Bedroom

WHAT ACTIVITY HAPPENS primarily in the bedroom, is an important element of fertility, and studies show that 60 percent of Americans don't get enough?

Believe it or not, we're talking about sleep, not sex. During the first half of Week 4 our goal is to turn our focus to this very pleasurable but undervalued part of our fertility regimen. Over the next seven days our goal is to determine our sleep needs and to find ways to enhance the quality of those healing zzzs in order to promote fertility.

In Chapter Three, we discussed how poor nutrition can disrupt reproductive hormone regulation. Guess what! So does poor sleep. So, let's get down to business and find out how our sleep stacks up in the fertility department.

Sleep

Sleep is a true casualty of our modern lifestyle. Beginning with the creation of artificial lighting, we have slowly chipped away at the human need for sleep, using the "extra" hours for work and leisure. According to polls conducted by the National Sleep Foundation, in 1960 average Americans reported sleep times of 8–9 hours a night. In recent polls the same group found Americans reporting seven hours of sleep time.

Much of what we know about sleep comes from hooking sleep lab subjects up to three different machines: an electroencephalogram (EEG), an electrooculogram (EOG), and an electromyogram (EMG), which measure the activity of brain waves, eye movement, and muscle tone, respectively. The data collected by these machines show that sleep happens in two distinct phases: NREM and REM sleep. In a typical night we experience 4–5 periods of NREM (Non-rapid Eye Movement Sleep) followed by REM (Rapid Eye Movement Sleep). When brainwaves associated with each sleep phase are viewed on an EEG the two phases look very different. The NREM brainwaves are slower but bigger in amplitude. During NREM sleep our eyes make slow, rolling movements, our muscle tone is more relaxed, and our threshold to outer sensory stimuli is high. During NREM sleep our blood pressure and respiratory rates are also slow. REM sleep is characterized by faster, shallower brainwaves and erratic blood pressure and respiratory rate. REM sleep is associated with dreaming since subjects awakened during REM sleep typically report extensive dream details. REM sleep is only present in mammals and some young birds while NREM is present in reptiles, suggesting a more primitive purpose for NREM sleep.

In fact, it is not clear why we sleep at all. Many hypotheses exist, suggesting behavioral, metabolic and even psychological reasons why humans sleep. What we do know, however, is that sleep has an enormous impact on our fertility.

The Sleep/Fertility Connection

Peaceful, abundant sleep is imperative for optimal fertility. Like many of the lifestyle factors that have an impact on fertility, sleep interacts with optimal fertility on a multitude of levels. From a physiological standpoint, the endocrine system is vulnerable to sleep loss, meaning that the regulation of our hormones, moods and metabolism is dependent on good sleep habits. It is also during sleep that the body repairs itself on a cellular level and sleep is important for healthy immune function. For this reason, researchers have become more and more interested in the phenomenon called "chronic partial sleep deprivation," and its impact on our physiological and cognitive function. This low-level sleep deprivation is related to fertility. When researchers surveyed a sample of women from sleep-challenged professions (flight attendants and night nurses) they found that 50 percent of these women reported irregular menstrual cycles, compared to 20 percent in the general population. (*Bisanti, 1996*)

The pituitary gland, known as a "master gland" because it controls the release of hormones from other glands in the endocrine system, is affected by sleep loss. The link between sleep and sex-hormone regulation may be mediated by the pineal gland, a tiny endocrine gland located in the center of the brain that acts as a biological clock and a "light-sensor." The pineal gland is made up of endocrine, nerve, and retinal (eye) tissues and one of its primary functions is to regulate the sleep/wake hormones melatonin (which promotes sleep) and cortisol (which promotes wakefulness) by sensing the patterns of night and day, or the circadian rhythm. The pineal gland's role in signaling the hypothalamus to produce sex hormone-stimulating factors is also presumably mediated by circadian rhythm. In one model for a potential interaction between sleep and fertility, pineal function is disrupted when sleep patterns are disrupted by insomnia, improper lighting conditions in the bedroom, travel/time zone shifts, or stress. This disruption impacts the hypothalamic-pituitary axis (HPA) with a resulting impairment of menstrual/ovulation/sperm production.

Another inherently harmful effect of sleep impairment on reproductive function stems from the relationship between sleep and our autonomic nervous system. During deep sleep our body's parasympathetic (rest and digest) activity is greatly increased. Sleep loss increases sympathetic hormone release, a condition of elevated physiological stress that down-regulates sex hormone function. Other metabolic functions affected by disruptions in the parasympathetic/sympathetic balance are appetite control and insulin metabolism, which may in turn contribute to fertility-reducing conditions like diabetes and obesity. Disruption of sleep can have a profound effect on our mental/emotional state as well. As little as one hour of sleep disruption over the course of several days is enough to impair cognitive function. More profound cognitive effects occur when sleep loss is chronic or prolonged, even resulting in depression.

Optimal Sleep for Fertility

The goal for optimal fertility is to first establish how much sleep we need and ensure that we are indeed getting the full amount, and second to improve the quality of the sleep we are getting. So how do we know how much sleep we need? Experts suggest that while 7.5–8 hours a night is the average amount of sleep adults need, they also admit that a majority of people require more than this amount. So we have to get personal here. Do you feel rested during daylight hours, without the use of artificial stimulants like caffeine? If you experience periods of drowsiness during the day, chances are you are not getting the sleep you need. There's really only one way to know whether you're getting enough sleep and that's to go to bed at least an hour earlier for one week and create a sleep journal—and that's exactly what's on this week's agenda (see the Sleep Journal on p. 131).

The beauty of this simple experiment is that it immediately points to the link between our lifestyle and our sleep habits. Did you experience a moment of panic at the idea of getting to sleep earlier? Perhaps the hour between dinner (a late dinner, of course, because you were at work or finishing up some errands) and bedtime is the time that you actually *get things done* like pay the bills, order groceries, shop for dining room furniture, or (heavens!) actually catch up and chat with your partner.

If you did panic, that's okay. Shifting sleep patterns is challenging but it can be done. We are born with an inherent wisdom regarding the amount of sleep we need but even as little babies the stimulation of daily life and interaction with others draw us away from our natural rhythms. There's a truism with babies that "sleep begets sleep." The more consistently a parent puts a baby down to nap, the longer the baby will nap. This is not because we're creating a lazy baby; it's because by soothing and calming the baby, and putting him down in a dark quiet place, the baby learns to let go of the stimulation of his day and to relax into sleep that's both nourishing and important for development. The truth is we're no different from babies. The more we allow ourselves to get overtired, the less we are able to relax and settle ourselves into sleep. Just as a baby can't recognize when she's overtired, we too lose the ability to notice that we're overtired. And since we don't have a mommy to enforce regular naps and make sure we're bathed and lotioned and snuggled into our jammies, we need to do this for ourselves, too.

Apart from how we feel, there's another indicator of sleep quality that we can use to see if our experiment is working. As discussed above, one of the first physiological shifts seen when someone is entering a state of sleep deprivation is elevated cortisol levels. Elevated cortisol can also result in a slightly elevated Morning Resting Heart Rate, or MRHR. As part of our sleep experiment, we will be taking our MRHR over the course of the next week to see if we notice any correlation between resting heart rate and sleep quality.

This is also a good point in our program to put the book down and tap your partner on the shoulder. If he or she has resisted the yoga or the nutrition weeks, there is absolutely *no excuse* for them to opt out of the "extra sleep" week. We suggest this jokingly, but with a grain of seriousness. Many of the exercises planned for the week are pleasurable but will be much more effective if there's no "peanut gallery" wooing you to chuck your sleep program for a late night of red wine and *Frasier* re-runs.

Please Note: The experiment in this chapter is designed to help us identify borderline sleep deficiency. If you suffer from insomnia, you should consult with your holistic practitioner and your physician to explore holistic and medical options for this condition.

Beth writes:

As I look back on the fertility journey, my sleep patterns were probably part of my fertility problems. Between working and graduate school, I would routinely wake up at 4 a.m. to either study or squeeze in a run. Frequent were the days that 10 a.m. found me longing for lunch and a nap. Even though I went to bed relatively early, waking each morning in the dark and spending the first hours of each day in artificial light was disruptive to my hormonal balance. Between early bedtime and naps I did manage to total an average of 7–8 hours of sleep per day. However, in retrospect, I recognize that my sleep pattern was symptomatic of an over-full schedule. Add to that the intense physical exercise and stress of graduate school and there's no surprise that my reproductive system was compromised.

Now, just coming off the sleepless months following the birth of my second son, Calvin, sleep is by far the most precious of my bodily functions. I have learned over time that I require a solid 8 hours of uninterrupted sleep. Ten minutes under and I'm cranky and in need of a caffeine infusion, and ten minutes over and my eyes are wide open and I'm chirping like a robin. Now I always ask my yoga students how many of them are getting enough sleep and, sadly, I rarely see a majority of the class raising their hands. Once aware of the importance of sleep for fertility they begin to examine not only their sleep patterns, but lifestyle factors like stress that may negatively impact their zzzzs.

Dream Symbols

Dreams have played an interesting role throughout history. They were often revered, feared or shrouded in mystery. Cleopatra was said to have had a dream that her lover Julius Caesar would be slain. Scientist Friedrich August Kekulé discovered that the structural unit of the benzene ring consisted of a ring of six atoms of carbon. The particular arrangement of the carbon atoms had been a mystery until 1865 when Kekulé had a dream in which he saw a chain of carbon atoms rotating in a circle, like a snake chasing its own tail.

Not all dreams are premonitions of future events, nor are they necessarily omens. Modern scientists might argue that dreams are nothing more than electrical currents in our brain firing while we sleep, which causes the creation of images or patterns. At PDtM, however, we feel dreams are much more than images in our head. They play an important role in our mental and spiritual well-being because they allow us to take a peek into our unconscious thoughts and patternings.

Sigmund Freud once said, "Dreams are the royal road to the unconscious." He believed that every dream was a wish from the unconscious that should not be ignored. Carl Jung studied under Freud but developed a different view of dreams, which eventually led to a major rift between the two dream theorists. Like Freud, Jung also believed in the unconscious; however, he didn't see the unconscious as animalistic, instinctual, and sexual; he saw it as more spiritual. He believed that dreams help us get to know our unconscious. They were not meant to mysteriously conceal our true feelings from the waking mind, but were meant rather to be a window to the soul. Dreams may hold solutions to problems we are facing in our waking life.

Jung viewed the ego as one's sense of self and how we portray ourselves to the world. Part of Jung's theory was that all things can be viewed as paired opposites (i.e. good/evil, male/female, or love/hate). And thus working in opposition to the ego is the "counterego" or what he referred to as *the shadow*. The shadow represents rejected aspects of yourself that you do not wish to acknowledge. It is considered an aspect of yourself which is somewhat more primitive, uncultured, awkward, and unaware. By writing down and trying to interpret our own dreams, we are getting to know more about our shadow self and those patterns which are otherwise hidden from our everyday view.

Tami writes:

It is Jung's theories on dreams that we utilize most at PDtM. Symbols that appear in our dreams are important because they tell us a bit about what's going on in our unconscious. I once filled my home library with books on dream interpretations, studying the various symbols and their corresponding meaning. What I quickly learned is that dream and symbol interpretation is best left to the dreamer, not the psychiatrist, not the best friend, and not a textbook. You are the one who can most accurately interpret your dreams.

Symbols not only appear in our dreams but can also appear while daydreaming or meditating. While teaching a class at PDtM I instructed the class to spend 10 minutes meditating on an object of beauty. When the 10 minutes were over, one student reported that she had a difficult time concentrating on her object of beauty because an umbrella image kept popping into her mind. I asked the student what this symbol meant to her and she said, "It symbolizes getting out of the rain." So, I probed further, "What does the rain symbolize?" The student felt that the rain was the tumultuous nature her life had been in since undergoing fertility treatment. She then reasoned that the umbrella was her ability to stop treatment and "get out of the rain" anytime she wanted. Although she viewed her fertility situation as being "out of her control," she then realized that she ultimately controlled her destiny by the decisions she made. This simple, in-class exercise became somewhat of an epiphany for her.

Not everyone has an epiphany each time they analyze their dream symbols, but the practice can be useful for self-study. In section two of this book we delve more deeply into self-study and you may find your dream symbols quite interesting as we begin to examine the thoughts and ideas that inform our beliefs about fertility. In the meantime, we've included a section in your sleep journal for any symbols that may surface during this 12-week journey.

Bedroom Feng Shui

Feng shui, pronounced "fung shway," literally means wind and water. It has its roots in how the ancient Chinese noticed the delicate interplay between these two forces of nature and their ability to shape our world and our environment. It's an ancient Chinese art of placement, known in the West as geomancy. This philosophy asserts that the arrangement of our surroundings can bring positive or negative energy to our environment and our lives. Feng shui dates back thousands of years to China, where the practice was applied to finding auspicious burial ground for royalty. This was believed to guarantee prosperity for future generations. Over time, the science and practice were developed and became a core belief of Chinese culture, involving a mix of religion, philosophy, mathematics, and astrology.

When reading about feng shui, you will come across the word "auspicious" a lot, which means good or favorable. Using the techniques of feng shui, you can make your environment more auspicious. This does not mean that bad things will never happen to you; it just improves your odds of experiencing good fortune.

Jeanie writes:

The Chinese are very concerned with circulation and energy flow. The energy flows in and around our bodies and we can use acupuncture, herbs, yoga, t'ai chi, and meditation to improve the way it flows. Energy also flows around us in our environment. We use feng shui to facilitate this flow and allow the energy to flow in its most natural and auspicious state. You may have had the experience of not liking the way your furniture was placed. Once you rearranged it, the room seemed to flow better; the energy flowed better, and your whole exis-tence improved that little bit. There are many simple things in our environment that can either help or hinder the flow of energy around us. Feng shui is the science of understanding and manipulating that information for our advantage. It is best known for helping you decide where to place objects in your home but is also used to determine the most auspicious time for planning certain events. When I became engaged, my mother spent two days drawing up and analyzing charts to determine whether our intended wedding day was auspicious or not. She determined that it was, and we married on that day.

- *The most auspicious room shape of the bedroom is square or rectangular. If your bedroom is L-shaped, you can hang love beads or crystals to make it into a rectangle or square.*
- *If the bedroom has a bathroom attached to it, lower the lid of the toilet and close the bathroom door whenever possible. The toilet is a place for drainage of turbid waste. We don't want any of the positive energy to drain and we do not want any negative energy to come back into our environment. Do not place the bed so that the head is on the opposite side of the wall from the toilet. If the situation is inevitable, place a mirror or reflective foil behind the headboard towards the wall to deflect any negative energy.*
- *Place the bed away from the doors and windows with accessibility to each side. Do not place the bed so that the feet are pointing to the door. This is considered a "coffin-like" position and as such may not be your best bet for fertility. If necessary, you can use crystals or a screen to separate your bed and the door. Vice versa, do not place your head towards the door either. This is believed to create "unseen danger" to the occupant. The most auspicious bed placement would be diagonally opposite from the door, not directly under the windows, with equal access from both sides of the bed.*
- *Do not store anything underneath the bed. Clutter under the bed inhibits good energy from flowing freely around the bed. Clutter is a big feng shui no-no as it blocks positive energy and accumulates "stale" energy. For fertility, good energy flow in the bedroom is essential.*
- *Mirrors or anything reflecting the bed in the bedroom have long been considered inauspicious, especially directly facing the bed or above the bed. Sleep gathers energy; mirrors tend to disperse that energy. Mirrors should not be placed in the bedroom. If they are, place them next to the bed.*
- *Overhead beams in the bedroom are said to send negative energy that splits the couple's harmony and romance. It's*

The science can get very involved and beyond the scope of what most people want or are willing to do, but the box above presents some general rules and guidelines so that you and your partner can improve your environment, your luck, and your fertility.

Ritual to the Moon

We recommend making this ritual a daily part of your journey toward parenthood. It is called Ritual to the Moon because it is meant to end the night, put closure to your day, and provide hope that tomorrow will be an even greater blessing to both yourself and those around you. As you continue to practice Ritual to the Moon, you may begin to see that best to avoid a room with overhead beams. If you have an overhead or structural beam in your bedroom, create a canopy over the bed to block out the negative energy coming directly down toward you.

- Television or any electronic devices such as electric blankets are not auspicious in the bedroom since they do not possess natural energy. If you have electronic devices in the bedroom, place a cover over them at night.
- Avoid sharp corners and edges in the bedroom; especially if they are pointing to the bed. Soften the edges by hanging a crystal in front of the edge or place a plant to absorb the negative energy.
- Waterbeds are not auspicious since the bed does not give stability. Water paintings and/or an aquarium in the bedroom is not auspicious either; water tends to make things soggy.
- Growing plants and flowering plants are to be avoided in the bedroom since they possess strong yang energy. Flowers create good yang energy but not in the bedroom. When present in a couple's

bedroom it can cause infidelity and disagreement. Do not hang pictures of other men or women in the room either. It's said this can cause affairs!
- A bedroom should be yin in nature; lighting and colors should be soft and subdued to create a calm and relaxed environment.

The following decorative items, symbols, and foods are considered auspicious for fertility:
- A Chinese Double Happiness sign under your mattress
- A pair of Mandarin ducks in the southwest corner of your bedroom
- Elephants
- Dragons
- Double Fish symbol
- Hollow bamboo
- Red paper lanterns
- Pomegranate
- Lychee fruit
- Longan fruit
- Lotus seeds

there are a number of changes that take place in your personality due to the inner reflection and self-study that occurs. It should be practiced every night just before bedtime. Hopefully, this will become a regular part of your evening not just during conception time, but long after you are holding that baby in your arms.

STEP 1: DUTY
Perform your typical evening rituals. Put your night clothes on, brush your teeth, wash your face, put your reading material down, unmake your bed, or do anything necessary in preparation for sleep.

STEP 2: ASAN

Sit in a meditative posture for at least five minutes and focus on the third eye, the point located just above the eyebrows in the middle of your forehead. Simply sit and observe the contents of your mind. Download data but remember, you are observing here, not judging.

STEP 3: CONTEMPLATION

Now that you have observed the contents of your mind, sit in contemplation. Ask what went well about the day and commend yourself. Then, ask what could have been better. How can you work on this or make it better tomorrow?

STEP 4: BREATHE

Take a series of long, slow inhales and exhales. As you inhale, imagine you are filling your body with fresh prana or life energy. As you exhale, you are getting rid of all the negative things you said, did, or felt that day. Inhale life, exhale death.

STEP 5: PRAY

Ask God or the Powers that Be to help you move forward in your journey with strength, grace, and ease. Ask for guidance, assistance, or anything you need at this time.

STEP 6: LOCK

Sitting in a cross-legged position, take your arms and place them behind your back. Grab opposite elbows behind you. If you cannot reach your elbows, grab your wrists. While maintaining this hold, take your chest down toward your legs. Hold the muscles around the perineum as if you are stopping the flow of urine. Pull the navel up and in. Take your chin down toward your chest. By doing this, you are engaging the energy locks in the body which seal in the good intentions, meditations, and prayers you have just created through your ritual.

STEP 7: RELAX

Get up from the floor and relax for at least five minutes. Find inspirational quotes to read in your bed, turn the lights off and just lay in bed, or listen to soft, relaxing music. This is your time to completely let go and unwind before bedtime. Remember, you have just completed a sacred ritual. This is not the time to turn on the TV only to be bombarded with negativity from the daily news or a horror movie. Nor should you be reading material that is not inspirational or uplifting. It's a good idea to keep a few meaningful books, some poetry, or a collection of prayers on your bedside table that you can leaf through while in this peaceful space. When you are finished relaxing, go to sleep.

Fertile Sex

On the surface, the issue of sex and fertility seems like a major no-brainer. As we learned so long ago in high school health class, sexual intercourse is the number one way to get an egg and a sperm to do their dance in the right place at the right time. Of course that's the same health class where we were also taught that it's very easy to get pregnant and that all it takes is one determined little sperm to seal the deal. Okay, well that was probably pretty sage advice for a group of 16-year-olds, but here we are, several million sperm later and still not pregnant. Gone is the hopelessly romantic idea that your child will be conceived in a moment of passion and that you'll be able to tell her that "you were conceived in Paris after a fabulous meal and a vintage-year Bordeaux."

Suddenly the baby-making sex doesn't seem so exciting and sexy any more. Disheartening would be closer to the mark. Or *compulsory*. Heaven help anyone or anything that stands between you and the sex act on days 10 through 16 of your menstrual cycle. Getting that sperm and egg together has become a mission for which work schedules, vacations, and social life are sacrificed. What used to be an afterglow is now ever so slightly tainted by the question "Was this the time?"

If it wasn't the time, and more weeks and months and even years of passionate moments come and go and no baby appears, three things commonly occur. The first is that most couples throw their hats into the ART arena. By this time, "boom-boom burnout" has set in and many couples may even be initially relieved that the "work" of procreation will be handed over to the professionals. Yet along with the relief, the medicalization of the baby-making process can bring a sense of loss. The dream of "natural" conception has ended and there may be trepidation about the medical journey that is about to begin. The names of the procedures, intra-uterine insemination (recently renamed from the even more heinous *Artificial Insemination*) and in-vitro fertilization (test tube babies!), underscore their distance from the biological acts of sex and conception. And finally, the gory details of the fertility work-up process can introduce new feelings of guilt or blame as elements of biological viability come into play. Suddenly a host of previously unknown particulars come to light about a partner's FSH levels, egg quality, and sperm counts. To pretend that this process of medicalization has no impact on our sex lives would be plain old denial.

The sex element of the infertility process has also become a staple for pop-culture as couples on *Friends, Sex in the City*, and even *Frasier* (remember Niles's Test-a-cool pants?) struggle to conceive. The standard cliché is the image of a woman, with thermometer in mouth, telling her harried husband that they have to *do it right now because she's ovulating!* Her partner manages to do his duty (wink, nudge) and everyone has a laugh at this *terrible* problem. That he (or she) should not be in the mood, or that—gasp—he should be unable to perform, is just not part of our cultural myth.

As women who have been there and done that (and done that and done that and done that), we know that there is often a different story than the one we see on TV. This is just one more of the many elements of the trying-to-conceive (TTC) process that make us feel isolated. While everyone else can laugh at the images presented in the media, if we are experiencing the same things in our own life and don't find them quite as funny, it can compound the sense of isolation that often accompanies the fertility journey. Sex is an important part of our lives and trying to conceive takes this fun, creative, loving experience and makes it feel like work. Worse yet, it makes it feel like work we're just not good at. So let's take a closer look at the importance of sex during ART—beyond the role of conception—and see if we can't demystify what makes sex "fertile" and how we can improve our overall sex life while trying to conceive or doing ART.

CHECKLIST FOR "FERTILE SEX"

During the process of trying to conceive, we have to have a lot of sex. We thought we'd check in with Dr. Laura Berman, author of *The Passion Prescription: Ten Weeks to Your Best Sex–Ever!*, to see if she had any suggestions for us on how to make the sex we have more conducive to conception. If you're currently doing IVF and feel that the sex act isn't for procreation any more, let us remind you of the number of babies we've seen at Pulling Down the Moon that were conceived during a period of "time off" from medical intervention. Here's our checklist:

When to "Do It"

Common sense suggests that for sex to be procreative, you have to get the sperm and the egg together in the right place at the right time. While we know where the right place is, the timing issue is still not completely clear. Conventional wisdom suggests that conception is more likely to occur at mid-cycle, when the egg has been released from the ovary, but there are actually *two* schools of thought on this topic. The first school emphasizes timing sexual intercourse with a woman's ovulation. Basal Body Temperature (BBT) charting is a great resource for understanding your body's fertility signals (changes in cervical mucous, shifts in cervical position, etc.) and teaches you how to identify your most fertile time of the month and time intercourse accordingly. More about BBT charting can be found in the Appendices. BBT charting can also provide an enormous amount of information about your menstrual cycle and potential cycle irregularities. For instance, you might learn that you ovulate earlier or later than day 14, or that you have a short luteal phase. However, students at Pulling Down the Moon often express that the process of taking and charting their BBT can be stressful and for many of them it becomes yet another element of fertility to obsess over.

On the flip side are the proponents of the strategy of "spreading the love," or having sex at least two times per week, every week—and relying on the odds that this will result in conception over the course of six months to a year. At PDtM we lean closer to this "spread the love" camp. There are also some good scientific reasons to consider the broader, twice-a-week approach. In a recent study published in *Fertility and Sterility*, researchers conducted ultrasounds on 63 women between the ages of 18 and 40 and found that 68 percent of them experienced multiple waves of follicle development. (*Baerwald*, 2003) Anecdotally, we have seen women conceive at PDtM who swear they did not have sex during their most fertile period but conceived none-the-less. There's a certain element of magic to the dance between egg and sperm that we prefer not to pigeonhole.

Beth's BBT "Confessions:"

I was a gung-ho BBT charter. As a matter of fact, I still have the BBT charts for Georgia, Jackson, and Cal. I learned a lot from this method—most importantly that I had a short luteal phase, that I ovulated quite late (day 21 of a 28-day cycle), and that my post-ovulation temperature rise wasn't very strong. This information allowed my holistic practitioners to suggest changes to a number of my health habits. The theory was that my body was too depleted to ovulate "on time" and once it mustered up the umph to ovulate, there was no energy left to sustain implantation. My Ayurvedic physician suggested that I change to a warming diet, improve my sleep, and reduce stress in order to strengthen my ovulation. As I made these changes I did see a shift in my luteal phase and a stronger temperature rise.

There was, however, a dark side to my BBT charts. The post-ovulatory temperature rise became a major focus in my life. After ovulation I would take my temperature two, three, maybe four times a day. Even though I was fully conscious of the fluctuation of body temperature at different times of the day, I could not get the thermometer out of my mouth. When the temp was high, I was happy, and if it dipped I was in tears. My husband had it with me and the thermometer. I can clearly remember hiding in my bedroom taking my temperature for about the ninth time of the day and my husband hearing the beep-beep-beep of the digital. I was busted!

I still laugh when I look at the BBT chart for my last baby, Calvin. It clearly indicates that my date of conception did not correspond at all with my ovulation as charted by BBT (and an ovulation predictor—I liked having back-up!). Throughout the first trimester, ultrasounds consistently measured him one week behind my ovulation date, suggesting that he was conceived a week later than I had thought. I have often wondered if I ovulated twice that month and he's here because I had recreational sex during a "non-fertile" time that I might have missed if I had only been trying at mid-cycle. Bottom line is that it's a mysterious dance that the sperm does with that little egg and we can never be sure when it happens.

Lubrication is Not Just a Good Idea...It's a "Fertile Sex" Law

For some reason, women tend to get a bit puritanical about sexual lubricants. Perhaps admitting that lubricant could be useful makes us feel like a failure, or brings up a sensitive issue with our partner. One Moon student recently expressed that she felt her husband would be insulted if she suggested that she needed lubricant, like he wasn't "turning her on" the way he should. Well, ladies, let us say right here, right now, that we've spoken with the experts and lubrication is not just something that improves how sex feels; it is a matter of life and death for the sperm that are on a mission to fertilize that ovum.

According to Dr. Laura Berman, here's the way it works. The more lubricated a woman is, the better. Sperm cannot survive in the typically acidic environment of the vagina. When a woman becomes aroused there's an increase of blood flow to the vagina which causes engorgement in the vaginal walls as well as externally in the labia. As there's pressure building on the walls of the capillaries lining the walls of the vagina, they begin to leak a kind of plasma—some comes from the cervix, some from bartholin glands at the base of the vagina, but the bulk of the lubricant comes from this engorgement, and the resulting lubrication changes the pH to a conducive environment for sperm survival.

Bottom line is that even if you feel you don't need it, a sperm-friendly lubricant can make the life of sperm much happier.

Are Some Positions Better Than Others for Conception?

Dr. Berman suggests that the most fertile positions are those that stimulate orgasm in the woman. A lot of ancient texts suggest that it is preferable for a woman to achieve orgasm *after* the man for sex to be procreative. According to Dr. Berman, this makes sense both for obvious reasons of pleasure, but also because there's a pooling area at the top of the vagina that the uterus dips down into after orgasm. When a man ejaculates, there's a pool of semen that the cervix can dip into and suck in the sperm.

However, Dr. Berman is not too hung up on the *order of operations*. If female orgasm comes first, the vagina will be nicely lubricated when ejaculation occurs. She suggests that female orgasm is important but certainly not necessary for a woman to conceive. However, if a woman is experiencing stress or anxiety about a loss of sexual response or inability to climax, she should seek help and support on these issues.

Dr. Berman also suggests that a couple end intercourse in missionary position as this position allows for the release of sperm deep in the vagina. As far as the age old question of standing on our head after sexual intercourse, our view at Pulling Down the Moon is that it's just as effective to put a pillow under your hips and relax. There's no scientific evidence that this improves the odds of conception but it certainly can't hurt.

Recognizing When There's a Problem

Dr. Berman acknowledges that sex can become a silent battleground during the fertility process. In fact, she sees a fair amount of patients in her practice who have come to her for assistance for this reason. She suggests that some signals that the problem may be reaching beyond "run of the mill" are:

- Arousal problems: if a woman is no longer able to reach orgasm; if she's experiencing dryness or lack of sensation or has low desire; if her partner is experiencing low desire, having erectile problems, trouble reaching orgasm or reaching orgasm too quickly.
- A change in sexual function, change in comfort level with each other sexually, or resentment of sex by one or both partners.

Chinese Sexology

One of the oldest sex manuals in the world is known as the *Handbook of Sex*, recorded about 5,000 years ago by the Yellow Emperor Huang Di. The book, written in conversation format between the Yellow Emperor and the Plain Girl, lays out the importance of proper sexual behavior, intimacy, arousal, satisfaction, and reproductivity of male and female. Books on Chinese Sexology, also known as Chinese Pillow Books, were used as marital aids by members of the imperial court and aristocrats. One of the most vital messages they present is the importance of a man's ability to satisfy the woman through techniques and observation. Although the manual was written thousands of years ago, the descriptions of the behavior and physiology are very similar to what was reported in *The Kinsey Reports: Sexual Behavior in the Human Male* (1948) and *Sexual Behavior in the Human Female* (1953).

Sex in ancient Chinese culture, was much talked about but through metaphors. They used terms such as Jade Stem (penis) and Jade Valley (vagina) to refer to the sexual organs in a poetic manner. Intercourse was alluded to as "love play of cloud and rain."

Importance of Female Satisfaction (Foreplay)

It's more difficult for the female to become aroused. According to Taoist sexual practice, from which most of Chinese sexual practice has been derived, it's very important that both partners be aroused prior to coitus. The male partner should take time and work on the female partner until she reaches the state of desire to have intercourse. As we all know, most of the time when the male has finished, the act is finished.

Erotic Partner Massage

This technique is used to enhance arousal and receptivity. In his book *Taoist Bedroom Secrets*, Chian Zettnersan divides the body into three regions. The primary zones are the most sexually stimulating; the lips, nipples, labia, clitoris, and tongue. The secondary zones are the earlobes, nape of the neck, low back, buttocks, and knees. The last zones, also called tertiary zones or neutral zones, include the pinky finger, the navel, toes, soles of the feet, and the openings of the nose and ears. The massage sequence starts with the *secondary zones*, then moves onto the *primary zones*, and finishes with *tertiary zones*.

Work your way around the body and enjoy all the stimulation. You can also incorporate "erotic kissing" with the massage. The Chinese considered erotic kissing as part of important sexual communication and unity of Yin (female essence) and Yang (male essence). Gentle touches can accommodate the erotic kissing. The touch should not be strong; the amount of pressure used is very light. The touch of the clitoris should be as light as a feather. This process can take as long as 20 to 30 minutes until the female partner is fully aroused.

Let's start the massage with *secondary erogenous zones*. The secondary erogenous zones are to be massaged from right to left in a *counterclockwise direction* (except for the nape of the neck), starting from the top.

- The earlobes: massage from right earlobe to left. In Chinese medicine, there are points in the ear that correspond to every part of the body. In fact, some acupuncturists treat all disorders only using the ear.
- The nape of the neck: this area is where the neck meets the shoulder. Massage gently in clockwise direction 72 times then counterclockwise for 72 times. This massaging is said to open all the channels in the body for Qi to flow more freely.
- Low back: the most important area is the small of the back to the tailbone. Massage in a counterclockwise direction.
- Buttock: make sure to get to the bottom of the crease, where the buttock meets the back of the legs.
- Inner thighs: massage gently in an upward fashion, counterclockwise.
- Back of the knees: in light strokes, again, counterclockwise.

When done, move immediately to the **primary zones**. All the primary zones are massaged, stroked, and/or kissed in a *clockwise* direction. The caressing of the primary zones start at the lips.

- Lips and tongue: in Chinese medicine, the lips are linked with the labia, both representing "openings" to the body.
- Breasts and nipples: the stimulation of the breasts is said to open the third eye. In Chinese medicine, the third eye is also known as upper Dan Tien, where Qi is stored and generated.
- Labia and clitoris: the genitals are related to the Heart organ in Chinese Medicine.

The Heart is also represented as Fire and the Spirit. Massaging this area is igniting a spark to start the Fire. Just as a fire must be carefully stoked and fed to become a blaze, the arousal of the woman's sexual organs requires finesse and perseverance.

According to Chian Zettersan, the tertiary zones do not have too much stimulatory effect unless the secondary and the primary zones are stimulated. The tertiary zones may not be what we normally consider erogenous zones, but Chinese medicine understands the subtle circuitry of the body. For example, the first tertiary zone to massage and stroke is the small finger (pinky finger). The small finger is connected to the Heart meridian, which can stimulate blood flow to the reproductive organs.

- Small finger: light stroking of the sides of the finger stimulates the Heart channel.
- Palms of the hands: all the acupuncture meridians or channels begin or end at the hands or the feet. Gently massage or stroke in a circular motion.
- Navel: very gently, massage this area 72 times clockwise and 72 times in a counterclockwise direction.
- Nostrils: these are also openings to the body, and they are connected with one of the five senses. As such, they can be sensitive, and kissing and stroking them can have an erogenous effect.
- Ear canal: blowing into your partner's ears is a well-known technique for inducing arousal.
- Soles of the feet: similar to the hands, the feet are connected to much of the body. The soles in particular are where the Kidney channel begins. As mentioned in the previous chapter, the Kidneys are the source of our reproductive essence.
- Big toe: the Liver Channel, which wraps around the genitals, starts at the big toe. Stroking, kissing and sucking on the big toe has been known to bring people to orgasm.
- Extra point: San Yin Jiao Point (four-finger length above the inner ankle bone). This is a meeting point for all three Yin organs of the lower extremities. Massage this point as a part of foreplay. Now, light the candles, turn on the music, and try these out!

While traditionally, Chinese sexology focused on the preservation of a man's Jing (semen) and longevity, this knowledge provides us with valuable information that we can use to increase both enjoyment and productivity of sex.

Traditional Aphrodisiacs

In Chinese Medicine, herbs that supplement Yang are considered to increase libido. Many of the herbs are foods eaten commonly on a daily basis.

- Walnuts: most nuts and seeds are considered good for fertility. Enjoy them as snacks throughout the day.

- Lyciium berries (aka Goji berries): in Asia, these berries have been long regarded as an anti-aging food. In OM, they are used to strengthen the Kidney and enhance fertility. Available in dried form, the berries make a great substitute to raisins.
- Cordyceps Sinesis: one of the most well-known Chinese herbal aphrodisiacs, cordyceps belongs to a rare fungus or mushroom family. Due to the herb's ability to build both Kidney Yin and Yang essence, the Chinese have regarded this herb as a major tonic to Chinese emperors for centuries. Cordyceps is also used widely to boost sexual energy and to increase the immune system. This can be made into a tea form for long-term consumption.
- Ginseng: the Chinese word for ginseng is *"ren shen,"* which literally translates as a "man root" because it looks like a human body. It is a powerful herb for strengthening Qi and has been traditionally used as a sexual tonic. Chinese ginseng contains compounds that may have effects on your body resembling those of certain sex and adrenal hormones. While it does not act as an immediate sexual stimulant, when taken long term it can enhance your sexual vitality. Ginseng can be taken in a tea form or the roots can be added to a soup stock to give "tonic" effect. Depending on the region of growth, Ginseng has different energetic properties. As with all Chinese medicinal herbs, ginseng can be harmful in the wrong circumstance and should only be taken with the advice and oversight of a trained practitioner of herbal medicine.
- Epimedium: in the West, this plant is known as "horny goatweed." As the name implies, this is known to have male hormone-like actions when taken. In OM, Epimedium is a herb to supplement Kidney Yang, and to treat impotence and infertility. Epimedium also has a boosting effect on the immune system. Usually used in a herbal formula with other ingredients, this herb is not to be taken long term. Be sure to consult a herbalist or an acupuncturist before taking this herb.
- Damiana: native plant to Central and South America, Damiana has been used as an aphrodisiac for men and women in Mexico, South America, and the West Indies for centuries. When ingested in tea form, Damiana increases both sexual desires and sexual performance in women and men. This herb is not recommended during pregnancy.
- Ashwagnadha: also known as Indian Ginseng, Ashwagnadha is used primarily as a strengthening tonic in Ayurveda. It treats infertility, impotence, sleep disorder, and aging. Not as expensive as Chinese or Korean ginseng, Ashwagandha is safe and effective. Usually prepared in a tea form with warm milk.
- Chocolate: the Aztecs referred to chocolate as the "nourishment of the Gods." Chocolate contains chemicals thought to affect neurotransmitters in the brain and a related substance to caffeine called theobromine. Chocolate contains more antioxidants (cancer preventing enzymes) than red wine. A guilt-free pleasure!

WEEK 4 ACTIVITY 1: KEEP A SLEEP AND DREAM JOURNAL

Over the course of one week, your assignment is to go to bed one hour earlier than usual. Upon waking, take your morning resting heart rate for one minute, using two fingers on the carotid artery and a clock with a second hand. Record the rest of the information, including what you remember about your dreams.

DATE & DAY OF THE WEEK	MONDAY	TUESDAY	WEDNESDAY	THURSDAY	FRIDAY	SATURDAY	SUNDAY
ASLEEP TIME:							
WAKE UP TIME:							
TOTAL SLEEP HOURS:							
HOW DID YOU FEEL ON WAKING?:							
MORNING RESTING HEART RATE							
ALCOHOL, CAFFEINE OR OTHER STIMULANTS?							
BEDTIME ROUTINE							
DREAMS							

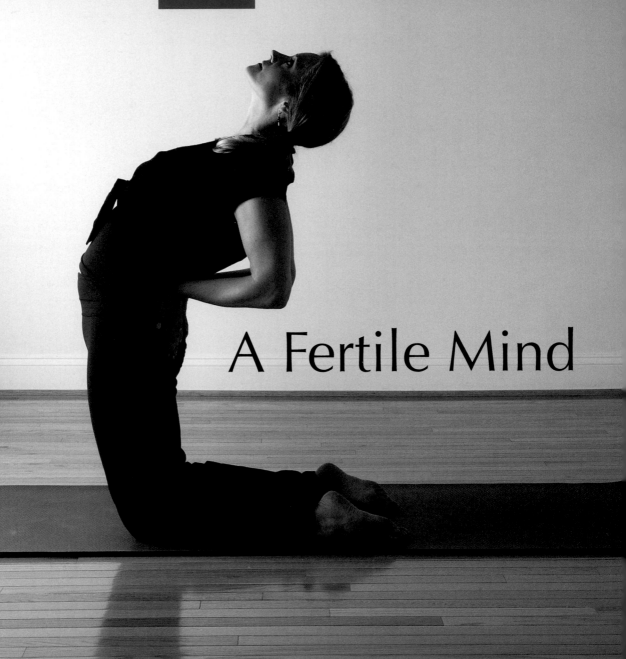

SECTION 2

A Fertile Mind

Strengthening the Letting-go Muscle

IN THE FIRST SECTION of this book, you were asked to look at some of the many ways you might enhance your fertility by engaging in certain practices for your physical body. Activities like eating more nutritiously, sleeping better, seeing an acupuncturist, exercising and doing yoga are practices that you will, hopefully, begin to take up to make yourself fully fertile. The way in which you adopt these practices will be very individualized. In other words, how and when you decide to eat, sleep, or do yoga might be very different from a co-worker who is also trying to achieve pregnancy. In yoga, when you begin the process of mindfully practicing things everyday to help you achieve physical, mental, or spiritual well-being it is called your *sadhana* or spiritual practice.

You might ask why nutrition, sleeping, or exercising would be considered spiritual practices. Caring for the temple of your body is a very important sadhana because the body is the only vehicle our spirit has to ride around in on this Earth. We'll talk more about your spiritual anatomy later in the book. For now, let's work on understanding why trying to have a baby can be so darn stressful. We think "Strengthening the Letting-go Muscle" is a good title for this chapter because in addition to adopting certain practices for fertility, there are, on the other side of the coin, some things that you will definitely need to give up. The process of letting go of quirks, attitudes, vices, disappointments, and negative thoughts is never easy. In truth, most of us will work our entire lifetime in an attempt to rid ourselves of those things that possess us.

The sacred texts of the *Yoga Sutras of Patanjali* call those things that we follow as a practice *Niyamas* (observances) and those that we restrain from doing our *Yamas* (abstentions). In order for life to be harmonious, it must be a balance of the two. There are many books out there today that interpret the Niyamas and Yamas and we recommend reading one of them if you are so inclined to learn more about this eight-limbed path.

In keeping with the spirit of these laws and becoming fully fertile, we will need to take up some new practices and let go of some of the old. You've heard it a dozen times before: out with the old and in with the new.

Let's begin this section by discussing some of the things on the fertility path from which you should try to abstain or let go of. The first and hardest thing you need to work on is letting go of some of your stress. Although some stress is completely unavoidable, fertility-related stress can and should be managed through practices such as yoga, meditation, breathing, visualizations, massage, or acupuncture.

Letting Go of Stress

When we ask our students at PDtM why they think they are having a hard time getting pregnant, the most common response is, "I'm too stressed out." This probably comes as no surprise to you as many of us face the daily struggles of increasingly demanding careers, competitive work environments, financial burdens, responsibilities at home, and the challenge of trying to find more time in a 24-hour day. We tend to work more, sleep less, eat quick and unhealthy meals, drink a lot of caffeine, pop pills, and relax less.

If you ask a medical doctor if stress causes infertility, she will likely say no, there is no concrete evidence that stress makes it difficult to conceive. In fact, the American Society for Reproductive Medicine has stated that "although infertility is a highly stressful experience, there is very little evidence that infertility can be caused by stress. In rare cases, high levels of stress in women can change hormone levels and cause irregular ovulation. Some studies have shown that high stress levels may also cause fallopian tube spasm in women and decreased sperm production in men."

Although doctors might not all agree that stress plays a major role in infertility, one thing cannot be disputed: the *process* of trying to conceive creates a great deal of stress. In one study, 112 women who were visiting their fertility clinic for a new course of treatment were given a psychiatric interview. Of these 112 patients, 40 percent had a psychiatric disorder with 23 percent showing signs of anxiety, 17 percent major depressive disorder and another nearly 10 percent exhibited dysthymic disorder, a less severe depression-like condition. Researchers concluded that women who visited an assisted reproduction clinic in anticipation of a new course of treatment had a very high rate of anxiety and depression. (*Chen* et al, 2004) Once a woman is depressed or anxious, her IVF success rate significantly declines.

When you look up the word stress in the dictionary, its most rudimentary definition states the following: importance, significance, or emphasis placed on something. By its very definition stress is subjective. We stress about that which we give energy to—that upon which we place emphasis. If we continually place emphasis on our inability to conceive, this inadequacy will become a stressor. The more energy and thought we give it, the more it grows. So, in essence, stress is determined by how much worth our mind places on something. This is an important factor in fertility because it illustrates how powerful conscious thought is on our physical and mental well-being. You've heard it before: energy follows attention.

If someone asked you to give a presentation about a topic you love in front of 100 people, how would you feel? For some of us, the mere thought of standing in front of a crowd that big would create an instant stress response in the body. For others, this type of performance might be considered the fulfillment of a life-long dream. In gaining a greater understanding of our fears and anxieties it is important to note that not all stressors affect people in the same way. In fact, the American Institute of Stress says a little bit of stress can, actually, improve productivity and performance in people.

In ancient days, upon meeting a tribal enemy or needing to battle a ferocious animal, the fight or flight response came in quite handy. This physiological response to stress had very important physical effects:

- Increases in heart rate, blood pressure, and breathing enhance the flow of blood to the brain improving the decision-making process.
- Blood also moves away from the stomach where it is not immediately needed for digestion and gets pumped to the large muscles of the arms and legs to provide more strength in combat or greater speed in getting away from the scene of potential peril.
- Blood sugar rises to furnish more fuel for energy as the result of the breakdown of glycogen, fat, and protein stores.
- Clotting occurs more quickly to prevent blood loss from lacerations or internal hemorrhage allowing us to fight for a longer duration of time.

So, to a large extent, stress is the body's way of adapting to life-threatening situations like when you are on a camping trip and see a brown bear in your tent licking its chops. The problem is that too many of us are in a constant state of "brown bearness." This is to say that once upon a time there was always resolution to our stress. You either got away or got eaten.

Today, our bodies still react with these same, archaic fight or flight responses that are now, not only unuseful, but potentially damaging and deadly. Repeatedly invoked, it is not hard to see how they can contribute to hypertension, strokes, heart attacks, diabetes, ulcers, neck, or low back pain and other diseases (American Institute of Stress, 2007). Many of these effects are due to increased sympathetic nervous system activity and an outpouring of adrenaline, cortisol, and other stress-related hormones. Put it all together and you can have physical symptoms of seeing that brown bear long after he has left your tent.

Accepting Stress

We love the classic example the Buddha once spoke of when he reached his enlightenment under the bodhi tree. As a sailboat went drifting by he noticed that if the sail was not pulled tight enough, it would not sail. If the sail was pulled too tight, it would break from the pressure and stress of the wind. This classic metaphor is a great symbol for how stress should be used in our lives—as a way to help balance—not to break. It should help us be more productive, not destructive, so we can more easily "sail" through life.

Whether you are just starting to "try" or have been working on conception for years, the process of getting pregnant can be stressful, even life-altering. We place ourselves under a microscope and, perhaps for the first time, begin to evaluate every aspect of our life from what we put into our bodies to how we handle disappointment. We also begin to question how we can bring another responsibility, another life into this world and still hold everything all together when we are already so stressed out ourselves.

So what, specifically, makes trying to conceive or going through fertility treatments so darn stressful? One of the major reasons we hear at PDtM is that unlike more tangible goals of working toward a promotion or saving for a new house, the pregnancy process is shrouded in mystery. No one can tell you exactly when the magic moment will occur. No matter how many diplomas hang on your wall, how much money sits in your bank account or how hard you "try," you cannot control how quickly your body will conceive a child.

Sure, you can be proactive in your quest. You can hire the best doctors, read everything there is to know on the internet, and modify your lifestyle habits but, for most of us, no matter how hard we work at it, we cannot predict when we will hold that child in our arms. For some of us, the very idea of not having control over the situation can itself create a great deal of stress and anxiety. Unlike other aspects of our lives where unpredictability is acceptable, we want to know that we can count on our body and its proper functioning to kick in when we really need it. When this doesn't happen as we expect, we begin to feel broken; first physically, then mentally, emotionally, and spiritually. That is why it is necessary to spend the next four weeks learning how to manage your thoughts and your attitudes. We like to call it, "strengthening the letting-go muscle" because one of the quickest ways to feeling better is by surrendering to the order of the universe and letting go of old, negative, and habitual patterns.

Stress versus Depression

For the purposes of your fertile health, you must understand that there's a big difference between feeling stressed and being depressed. With 40 percent of infertility patients experiencing stress or anxiety at some point in their treatment, it is easy to see how stress might eventually lead to depression. According to the National Institute of Mental Health,

30 percent of women are depressed. Just think about how staggering that number is—that's nearly one in every three women! In addition to affecting our mental well-being, depression is not good for our physical health either. Studies show that depression will be the second largest killer after heart disease by the year 2020. Researchers are now finding that when the body is under stress or depressed it produces certain chemicals that can cause inflammation in the arteries over time, thus contributing to coronary artery disease. In addition, being depressed may mean the body's stress response is working overtime or is over active which can increase the risk of heart disease.

Here's another interesting statistic. According to a survey by the National Mental Health Association (NMHA), 41 percent of depressed women are too embarrassed to seek help for their distress. We hope that by the mere fact that you have picked up this book, you care enough about yourself and your fertility to recognize when you might need professional help regarding your mood swings, anxiety, sleeplessness, or depression.

The Value of Psychotherapy: Yes, It's a Holistic Practice

Each of us has probably experienced a headache at some point in our life. Most of us, at the onset of the pain, simply pop a pain reliever and plan to feel better in 20 minutes or so. How many of you go the next step and actually wonder why you have the headache in the first place? When you get a headache, do you reach for your forehead wondering if you could be coming down with something? Do you think about what has brought you to that very moment and analyze your stressors from the day? How about your neck and shoulders? Are they stiff or tight? Is the pain coming from muscular tension? How much sleep did you get the night before? Maybe that's the culprit. Have you had your eyes checked lately? This could all be vision trouble.

You see, it is much easier to pop a pill and mask the pain rather than try to pinpoint the root cause. Now you might think that headaches are a trite example, but in fact, we should be trying to find the root cause for all our suffering from headaches to depression to why we are not ovulating. When a healthy woman stops menstruating it is often due to diet and exercise, eating too little or exercising too much. Often overlooked in treating infertility are the stressors that might be inviting these types of conception—inappropriate lifestyle habits.

In a pilot study of 16 women who had hypothalamic amenorrhea, researchers found increased levels of cortisol, the stress-related hormone, in their bodies. Conversely, (fertile) women who were ovulating normally did not have increased cortisol levels. The group with amenorrhea was divided into two groups. One group received cognitive behavioral therapy for 20 weeks, while the other group was merely observed. An impressive 80 percent of the women who received therapy started to ovulate again, compared to only 25 percent of those just being observed. Two of the women became pregnant two months after receiving the behavioral therapy. (*Berga* et al, *2003*)

Reducing stress through psychological intervention could restore ovulation in women whose ovarian function has previously been impaired. The study suggested that a lot of small stressors that might seemingly have little impact on reproductive health can play a major role in causing anovulation. Although it has been generally accepted that failure to ovulate is usually caused by energy deficits from excessive exercise and/or under-nutrition, researchers are now asking why women undertake such behaviors. Often dieting and exercise are ways of coping with psychosocial stress and such stress is often increased in women who do not ovulate. Studies also show that women with hectic jobs face the highest risk, and are often in denial about the stress in their lives. Lifestyle factors and their contribution in determining overall health and fertility can no longer be overlooked.

When a woman stops ovulating and wishes to get pregnant, her doctor will generally put her on ovulation-inducing medications. These medications can be costly and the patient may experience side effects. A woman may also be at greater risk for ovarian hyper-stimulation and conceiving multiples. Holistic practices that help reduce stress should be appropriate first steps in fertility treatment before drug therapy interventions are prescribed. Since holistic therapies are mind/body medicines, we would be remiss if we didn't suggest that you check in with yourself periodically to determine how you are feeling mentally and emotionally. If you think you might benefit (even slightly) from talking with a therapist, call your local fertility clinic and ask them for the name of a mental health care provider who understands fertility-related issues. Studies point out that many women rely on their spouse and families when they are feeling upset about their fertility-related issues rather than seeking help from a professional because they just don't know where to turn. They also worry about costs or have concerns about being perceived as "crazy" or having the inability to cope. Some clinics, like Fertility Centers of Illinois, offer a few free visits to their psychologist for those women who are patients. Make sure you check into all resources available to you and wear your therapy sessions as a badge of honor.

What We've Learned

So let's re-emphasize a really important message of this section. You need to explore both your physical and your mental well-being while trying to conceive. Depressed women have lower conception rates. Psychotherapy can help increase pregnancy rates by eliminating stressors and thus lowering cortisol levels which could inhibit ovulation. In addition to seeing a therapist, visit a holistic center that specializes in fertility to feel like you are taking some control back into your life. You will feel supported by your practitioner, learn lifestyle habits and receive therapies appropriate for fertility in the process. In the end you will feel better physically and often, through the process of self-study, begin to understand some of the root causes of your stress or anxiety.

WEEK FIVE ACTIVITY 1: MOOD ELEVATION

Your assignment this week is to practice and learn the following mood-elevating yoga practice. These postures, when done regularly, focus on opening your heart chakra, decreasing stress, and bringing positive energy into your body. Do this practice whenever you are feeling sluggish, down in the dumps, or unable to get out of bed.

Mood Elevating Practice

You can begin this practice on its own or, as time allows, start with 3 rounds of Moon Salutations as described in Chapter 1.

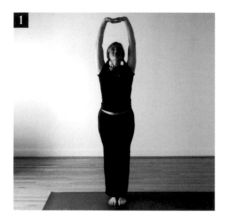

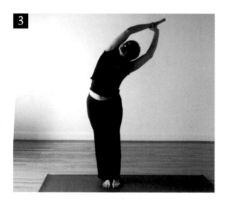

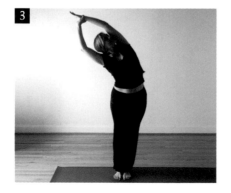

• *Ardha Chandrasana*

1. Inhale and lift your arms up over your head, turning the palms up to face the ceiling.
2. Stretch long, even lifting onto your tiptoes.
3. Grab your right wrist with your left hand. Exhale, take your hips to the right and your arms to the left. Hold for 5 breaths. In this posture you want to look like the crescent shaped moon shining in the evening sky.
4. Inhale and come back to center with your arms
5. Exhale and take your left wrist with your right hand. Lean to the right and stretch the left side of your body. Hold again for 5 breaths.
6. Come back to center.

Repeat this sequence 2 more times.

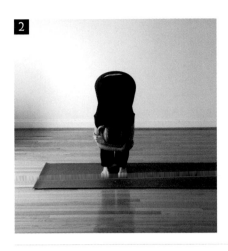

- *Uttanasana*
1. Place your feet hip-distance apart.
2. Hold opposite elbows and bow forward. Hold for 10 full breaths.

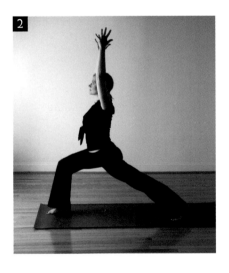

- *Virabhadrasana I Variation*
1. Take your right foot forward and step your left leg back.
2. Bend your right knee so it aligns with the top of the right ankle. Come onto the ball mount of your left foot and raise your arms up alongside your ears. You can arch your back a bit and open your heart if it feels okay for your body. Hold for 5 breaths.

Repeat on the other side with the left foot forward and the right leg back.

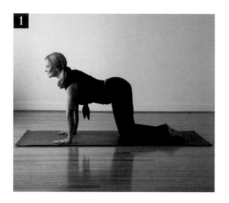

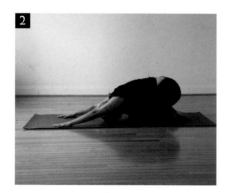

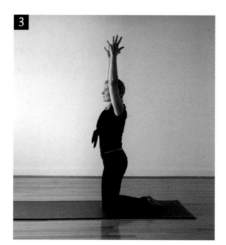

• *Happy Child Sequence*

1. Place your hands under your shoulders and your knees beneath your hips. Sink your chest without collapsing your shoulders. Arch your back slightly but keep the belly firm. Take an inhale in this posture, called "Table."

2. Exhale and move your stomach toward your thighs and your forehead to the ground in Child Pose (Balasana).

3. Inhale and lift your body off your legs and your arms upward alongside your ears.

4. Exhale back into Child Pose. Now you are back at step 1.

Repeat this sequence of four postures at least 5 times.

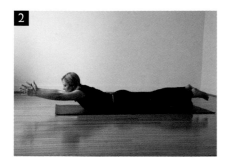

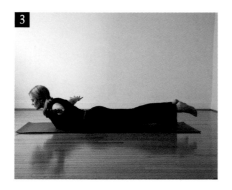

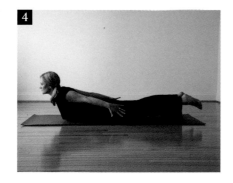

• *Salabasana (Locust) Series*

1. Lay on your belly (unless you are stimulating, bloated, or feel uncomfortable in doing so).
2. Inhale and lift your feet and hands off the ground by using the muscles in your abdomen and low back. Only your stomach will be on the ground with the legs touching at the thighs, knees, and ankles. Look straight ahead and allow the neck to be soft. Hold for 5 breaths and then release on an exhale.
3. Inhale again and lift up, keeping your arms and legs lifted. This time move your hands out to the side in a "T" position. Hold for 5 breaths and release on an exhale.
4. Finally, lift on an inhale and move your hands behind you so that they are alongside your body, keeping your legs lifted all the while.
5. Exhale and release your arms and legs. Now rest for a few breaths by making a pillow for your head with your hands.

Repeat this Salabasana sequence 3 times.

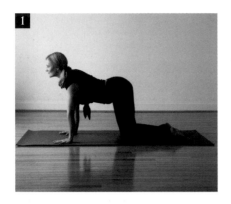

• *Downward Facing Dog*

1. Place your hands on the mat, shoulders' width apart.
2. Exhale and bring your hips up toward the ceiling in an inverted "V" shape. Straighten the knees as much as your hamstrings permit and press your heels toward the mat. Hold for 5 breaths.

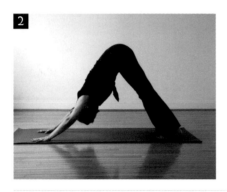

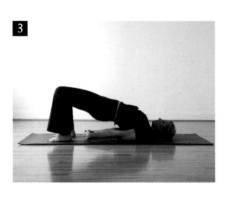

• *Setu Bandhasana (Bridge)*

1. Roll over onto your back and place your feet hip-distance apart and flat on your mat. Point the toes forward so that your feet are parallel to one another.
2. Inhale and lift your hips up toward the ceiling. Curl your shoulders toward each other on your back and, if your hands are available, clasp them together and use this leverage to move your hips and navel up higher toward the ceiling.
3. Hold for 10 inhales and exhales and then release.

Repeat 2 more times.

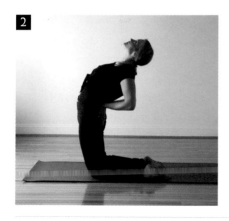

2

- **Ustrasana (Camel)**
1. Kneel on the floor with the tops of your feet flat and toes pointing behind you. Keep the thighs together. Knees and feet can be comfortably separated.
2. Rest the palms on your hips, lift the ribs, exhale and then curve the spine backward toward your feet. Look up toward the ceiling if it feels safe for your neck. Hold for 3–5 breaths and then rest by simply sitting on your heels.

Repeat Camel 2 more times.

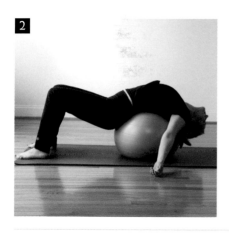

2

- **Supported Backbend**
This pose is contra-indicated for those with neck pain or injury.
1. If you have a large exercise ball like the one pictured, sit on it and then gently roll it under your sacrum so that it supports your low back. Melt your spine onto the ball and let your head and neck release.
2. Take your arms out to the side and simply breathe, focusing on the sounds of your inhales and exhales. Stay as long as you like.

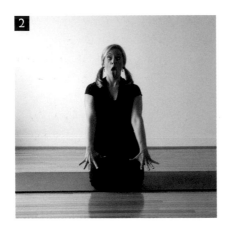

• **Simhasana (Lion)**

You might want to practice this one alone as you will you look quite funny doing it!

1. Sit on your heels with your spine nice and straight. Tighten the muscles of your face and stick your tongue out toward your chin as far as you can. Simultaneously, lift your brow and cross your eyes so that they are looking between your eyebrows or at the tip of your nose.

2. Stretch your arms out in front of you and open the fingers wide. Growl like a lion if you like. Hold the posture for a few breaths while breathing through the mouth.

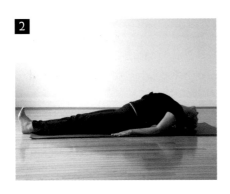

• **Matsyasana (Fish)**

1. Lie on the floor with your arms alongside you with a slight bend in your elbow.

2. On an exhale press your arms into the mat and arch the body back by lifting the chest and neck. Come onto the crown of your head and let it rest on the ground. Stay for 5 breaths.

3. To come out of the posture, push your forearms into the ground and lift your head first, thus allowing you room to straighten your back.

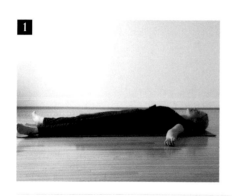

• *Janu Sirsasana (Head to Knee Pose)*

1. Sit down and extend your right leg forward.
2. Bend your left knee and take it out to the left side while bringing the sole of your left foot to the inner right thigh.
3. Exhale and bow forward by hinging at the waist and grabbing either the shin or ankle. For a more restorative posture, use a prop, like the bolster shown or a pillow, and rest your head on your prop. Hold the posture for 10 breaths.

Repeat on the other side by extending the left leg forward and bending the right knee.

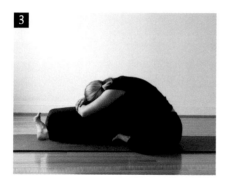

• *Savasana (Corpse)*

1. Lie on your back, letting the feet flop open and the arms to rest out to the side.
2. Dissolve into the earth and stay as long as you like.

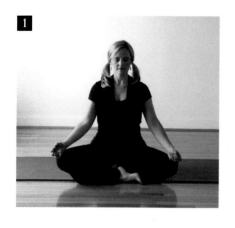

• *Meditation*

1. After you have completed your savasana, sit quietly in a comfortable cross-legged seated position for at least five minutes.
2. State an intention or say a prayer to lock in the positive and enlivening energy you have just created through your practice.

The Breath of Happiness

Finish your practice with the Breath of Happiness sequence pictured below. These postures all flow together quickly with the breath. Imagine your arms are moving constantly, like you are conducting an orchestra. Your knees simply bend and straighten with the movement of the arms. When the arms are up, the knees are straight. When the arms are moving downward, the knees are bending. The breath is simply three forceful inhales through the nose followed by one long exhale through the mouth at the end while vocally saying, "Ha." Say this very loudly and quickly. Get rid of all that pent-up frustration and anxiety.

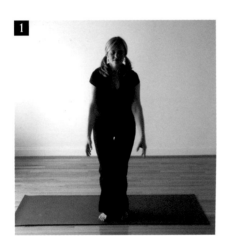

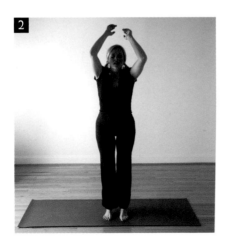

1. Starting position with neutral breath.
2. Lift up onto your toes and bring your arms overhead. Inhale quickly and forcefully through the nose so that you can hear it.

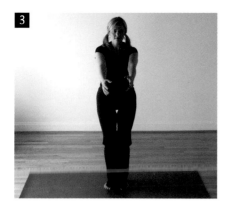

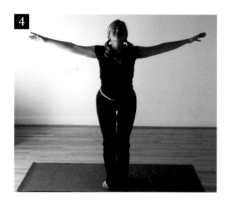

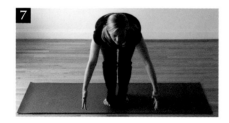

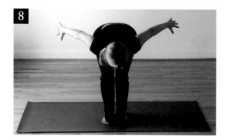

3. Bring the arms down and slightly bend the knees. Suspend the breath.
4. Forcefully inhale through the nose again while the arms reach out to the sides and the knees move toward straightening
5. Bring the arms back through the center while suspending the breath again.
6. Reach skyward again with the arms and take your third and final inhale.
7. Sweep the arms down toward the floor. When the fingers brush the floor exhale forcefully and say very loudly and quickly "Ha."
8. Let the head drop completely and the arms extend as far back as possible. Now sweep the arms back up toward the ceiling and begin this sequence all over again.

Seven Restorative Yoga Postures to Know and Love

The mood elevating practice and the breath of happiness may cause you to feel more energized and is not the best option when you are restless, anxious, or suffering from insomnia. In those cases, refer to the restorative yoga practice pictured below. These postures are also useful during ovarian stimulation time when you might feel bloated or distended. Additionally, the restorative practice is a good choice after both your retrieval and transfer during an IVF cycle.

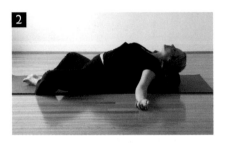

- **Supta Baddha Konasana (Supine Bound Angle)**
1. Bring the soles of your feet together and allow your knees to fall apart.
2. Lie down on your back or on a bolster and let your arms rest alongside your body. Stay here as long as you like, listening to the sounds of your breathing.

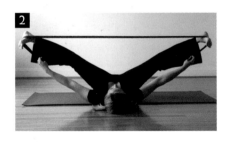

- **Supta Padangusthasana Variation (Reclining Big Toe Pose)**
1. Lie on your back and press the soles of your feet onto a yoga strap or rope.
2. Lift your legs up and then out, holding onto the rope for traction and support. As the muscles begin to relax, release more tension from the strap. Stay here as long as you like.

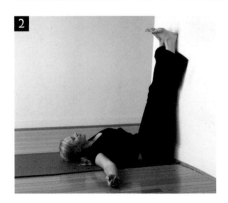

- **Viparita Karani (Legs Up the Wall Pose)**
1. Find a sturdy wall and sit sideways so that your hips are smack up against the wall.
2. Now lower onto your back and swing your legs up the wall for support. Flex your feet and extend your arms out to the side. If you have a bolster or blanket you can use it as a prop underneath your hips for added lift.

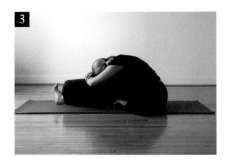

• Janu Sirsasana (Head to Knee Pose)

1. Sit down and extend your right leg forward.
2. Bend your left knee and take it out to the left side while bringing the sole of your left foot to the inner right thigh.
3. Exhale and bow forward by hinging at the waist and grabbing either the shin or ankle. For a more restorative posture, use a prop, like the bolster shown or a pillow and rest your head on your prop. Hold for 10 breaths.

Repeat on the other side.

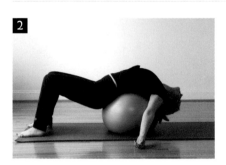

• Supported Backbend

This pose is contra-indicated for those with neck pain or injury.

1. If you have a large exercise ball like the one pictured, sit on it and then gently roll it under your sacrum so that it supports your low back.
2. Melt your spine onto the ball and let your head and neck release. Take your arms out to the side and simply breathe, focusing on the sounds of your inhales and exhales. Stay as long as you like.

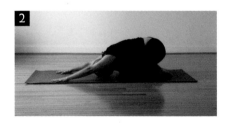

• Balasana (Child's Pose)

1. Start in Table Pose, on all fours with your hands under your shoulders and your knees beneath your hips.
2. Exhale and move your seat to your heels and your head to the floor.

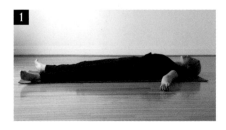

• Savasana (Corpse)

1. Lie on your back, letting the feet flop open and the arms to rest out to the side.
2. Dissolve into the earth and stay as long as you like.

Identifying and Eliminating Your Stressors

Dr. Esther M. Sternberg, physician and scientist, writes:

For so many thousands of years, popular culture believed that stress could make you sick, that believing could make you well. And people believe what they feel. But scientists need evidence. And there really wasn't any good, solid scientific evidence to prove these connections. Nor was there a good way to measure them. And scientists only believe what they can actually measure. Once scientists and physicians believed that there was a connection between the brain and the immune system, you could then take it to the next step: that maybe there is a connection between emotions and disease. Between negative emotions and disease, and positive emotions and health. And we can then say, okay, maybe these alternative approaches that have been used for thousands of years—approaches like meditation, prayer, music, sleep, dreams—all of these approaches that we really know in our heart of hearts really work to maintain health...maybe there is a scientific basis for it. (Sternberg, E. www.nlm.nih.gov. Online video—Celebrating American Women Physicians).

For years at PDtM we have been defining fertility as "the ability to grow," in all aspects of life, not just fertility. It is the ability to flourish in your relationships, your marriage, on the job, and with your career. If we begin to believe deep inside ourselves that we are fertile by its very definition, we can more consciously move away from the infertility stressor and move toward greater healing, personal growth, and happiness.

In order to achieve these types of positive results, you need to look at what kinds of stressors might be sticking in your craw because stress exists in many shapes and sizes. As we learned in the previous chapter, learning how to isolate the root cause of stress is a very important step in maximizing your fertility. So what are some of the fertility stressors and how do we recognize them? How do we know that what we are experiencing is completely normal and we're not as crazy as we think? Once identified, how do we eliminate these stressors? To help you answer these questions, we have included some commonly heard stressors from our classes at PDtM. When you are finished reading about them, ask yourself if any resonate for you. If so, make a note and commit to doing the corresponding exercise. That's it. That's your complete assignment for this week. Find your stressor, recognize it in yourself, and then work to eliminate it. It's okay if more than one of the stressors is present in your life. You can try many or all of the exercises to soften them if you like. You will probably discover this is not an all-inclusive list of stressors. You may have some that are very unique or particular to your specific situation. That's fine—go ahead and write them down. There is a general exercise at the end of this chapter that can be used for anything. Remember, we are looking for root causes of our stressors so let's get started.

Stressors of the Modern Day

For all the good things modern-day technology affords our society it has equally brought with it a great deal of additional work and stress. How many times a day do you find yourself answering "urgent" emails? We have to have things *now*: email me, fax it over, overnight that, call my cell, have a messenger deliver it.

Want to see true stress in action? Just go to the airport on a random Wednesday, the busiest travel day of the week, and you will see a great snapshot of stress in our modern-day world. Cell phones are ringing, computers computing, mobile email devices scrolling, backs and shoulders are breaking and flights are being missed. When travelers are not actively engaged in some sort of physical or mental stimulation, they are standing in line at fast food establishments and coffee shops or "chowing" down a meal before their flight boards.

Like it or not, most of us have hard-wired our internal computers to be "on" 24/7. There is simply not enough stillness in life to counterbalance all the activity, so the teeter-totter of life gets stuck. Ironically, the more we crave peace, the more elusive it becomes. Not only does this type of hectic lifestyle produce stress for the mind, it also creates stress in the physical body and can, ultimately, lead to sickness, anxiety, or even depression.

What most of us don't realize is that by living life at such a frenetic pace, we start to forget how to relax. Now this may sound ridiculous, but think about how stress affects the body. You will recall that stress releases adrenaline, cortisol, and other substances into the body like endorphins. Adrenaline creates a charge and endorphins are the same substance that create a "runner's high" in athletes. After a while, the body begins to crave these substances and we feel a bit sluggish without them. How many of us go on a vacation from work and discover it takes us two or three days just to unwind from the stresses of the week? We get this weird feeling like we should be doing something.

Modern-day stressors can indirectly affect your ability to maximize conception because you carry your "charge ahead" mentality into the world of fertility. You start on the treadmill of fertility and you simply cannot get off. What happens when we spend too much time on a treadmill or go too fast? We eventually just get plain old exhausted. There is a fine line between being persistent in your search for parenthood and being obsessive. Although persistence in trying to conceive almost always pays off in one way or another, having fertility occupy your every waking thought places your stress emphasis on something you currently have limited control over. It can become mentally and physically exhausting. Once again, energy follows attention. The more you emphasize your fertility the more it will emphasize you.

We have learned through our classes at PDtM that many women who can identify with this kind of behavior often describe themselves as "type A," well-educated, over-achievers. If you are hard-wired in this way, you need to learn how to shut down your computer periodically and reboot your thought process. It can be very therapeutic to stop dead in your tracks, to reorganize and change your momentum.

Here is a visualization you can try to help get you started with the process of letting go of stress. Find at least 5 minutes each day to practice this technique.

WEEK 6 ACTIVITY 1: REDUCING MODERN-DAY STRESSORS

Find a comfortable meditative position. This might be on the floor with your legs in a cross-legged position. It might be in a chair or leaning up against a wall for support. It is not lying flat on your bed because you may fall asleep and will lose the value of practicing this visualization.

Begin by taking a great big inhale through your nose until it completely fills your lungs. At the top of the inhale, hold your breath for three seconds. Then, release your breath through the mouth saying "Ahhhhh" out loud until all the air is expelled from your lungs. Repeat this process two more times. Now, return to normal breathing.

In your mind's eye, begin to picture all of your modern-day stressors as words or phrases on a white erase board. Data dump all of them onto your imaginary board and feel your mind begin to empty. Remember to include everything and anything on your mind even if it's things like grocery shopping, boss is an idiot, no money to fix car, call Kelly back, finish five-year trend analysis, etc. Now visualize all of your stressors out of your head and as words on the board. Take an imaginary eraser and begin to remove the words or phrases from your board one-by-one. Where there was once clutter on your board, notice that it is now white, clean, and blank. Once all of the words are gone, look into the emptiness of your cosmic dry erase board. Focus on the clean, white board. Notice the feeling of peace it creates inside of you. You are consciously wiping your slate clean. Spend at least five minutes focusing on your white board through this visualization.

Stressors from Friends and Family

It's so interesting to look at our culture and see that even though we have become increasingly progressive in our attitudes toward women and their roles in society, there is still a prevailing expectation that we should get married and have children. The societal expectation is that married couples should have children, carry on the family name or leave their living legacy. In fact, it might be perceived as somewhat "peculiar" if a married couple does not have children. We find ourselves contemplating the very reason why: she's too career-driven, they can't afford it, he's too selfish, their marriage is in trouble, they must not be able to have them.

Like it or not, we have been conditioned from long ago to believe that a woman's job is to keep those home fires burning, and that means having children. Whether the pressure to conceive comes from your mother-in-law, your best friend, or the women in your book club, it can create awkward conversations and a great deal of stress. Unfortunately, there is not a lot that we can do about how our society is conditioned from the past, but there is something we can do about how we handle the stress put on us by our mother-in-law, Aunt Mary Ann, or our best friend. Your option is two-fold: either politely ask them to mind their own business and be sensitive to the status of your fertility, or change your attitude and anticipate that people will say and do things that are, quite honestly, inappropriate. This is human nature.

Along these lines, Tami always tells this story as related to her by her guru, Goswami Kriyananda. If you own a cat, expect that the cat will scratch you. If you pet a snake, know that the snake might bite you. If you stand behind a horse, anticipate that the horse will kick you. And, if you are around human beings, be certain that they will "tongue" you. You see, no matter what physical form we take, we can never really get away from our own true nature. A cat's nature is to scratch, a snake to bite, a horse to kick, and people will say things that might hurt you or be inappropriate. It is their nature but, if we learn not to upset kitty, not to pet a snake, to stay in front of a horse and not behind, and to transcend the negative comments made by people, the pain will be much more tolerable. Once you practice this method, you will find it becomes second nature and the comments made by others will not "tongue" you in the least because you will realize that they just can't help themselves.

Epictetus, the Greek philosopher, said the world is divided into two realms: the things we cannot control and the things we can control. In the realm of things we can control, there is only one thing—our mind. We cannot control what other people do or say, but we can control how we react to what they do or say. Imagine that you are encased in a protective Teflon bubble and nothing can stick. We are not suggesting that you ignore these poisonous stressors, rather become immune to them over time by using your non-reactive behavior as your own form of immunity.

WEEK 6 ACTIVITY 2: REDUCING STRESSORS FROM FRIENDS/FAMILY

If you are feeling fertility stress from friends and family, it could be they are feeling an equal amount of stress from you. They may deliberately be avoiding certain conversations, or have guilty feelings about having children when you do not. In order to make all of you feel better, think about hosting a Fertility Summit at your home.

The first thing you will need to think about is your invite list. It is a good idea to invite everybody in your life who you think will benefit *you* in the long run. This may mean your list will include some folks you don't even like right now. It means inviting people who have been supportive of your fertility journey, those who have not, and those who don't even know. It is best to send the invitations by email or snail mail. Calling everyone just leaves you open to conversations best left for the Summit.

The actual Summit can be as elaborate or simple as you like. You could host a four-course dinner party or just ask people to come for a cup of tea. Allow time for everyone to gather, eat or drink and then begin the actual Summit. Start by telling your story: "As many of you know, John and I have been trying to get pregnant for quite some time now. We thought it would be easy but are finding that it is much more difficult than we had planned. Here's what we are currently doing." Then, proceed to tell your guests what you truly want them to know and understand. If you don't mind them asking you questions about your fertility, tell them so. If you do mind, ask them to be mindful of your feelings. The most important thing to do at the Fertility Summit is to reduce the stress you feel from your friends and family and to present your story from a place of strength rather than weakness. This is not a time to be crying "poor me," to get overly emotional, or start pointing fingers at people. It is a time for you to update them on your struggle and to tell them how you feel about it in a way that does not make your guests feel guilty, burdened, or sorry for you. Tell your friends and family that you are opening up about your experiences because they all mean a great deal to you and you need their love and support right now. In order to approach this from a point of strength, make sure you speak about two or three good things that have happened to you as a result of your difficulties with conception. Maybe you have a greater appreciation for life or a stronger relationship with your spouse. Think about it and make sure you share it.

Some of you may not want to open up about your wanting to become pregnant. Spend a few days and meditate on the reason why. If, after your meditation, you still feel strongly that you do not wish to expose yourself in this way, then don't. Have a pretend Fertility Summit. Stand up in front of a mirror and imagine you are telling your friends and family everything they ever wanted to know about your conception woes. Better yet, tape record yourself and play it every time you feel hurt by one of them. They may never hear it, but it will be therapeutic for you to play it.

The Jealousy Stressor

Each of us who has gone through the process of trying to have a child can probably relay a story about an insensitive friend or the "fertile Myrtle" down the street who never had any trouble getting pregnant and now has goo-gobs of kids. This group of friends find themselves knee-deep in diapers, baby clothes, and PTA meetings; usually complaining a lot about how busy they are and how their selfish lives have been transformed since they had children. Never realizing how alienating their lifestyle and comments can be, you may find yourself on the outside looking in as they plan play dates together and trips to the zoo without you. It doesn't matter, though, even if they invited you, you probably would decline. After all, they're all pushing strollers and you don't want to be the fifth wheel.

So what do you do when you are the last one in your social group without kids? How should you feel when everyone around you is getting pregnant and you're still "trying?"

We run a lot of classes at PDtM and it is very educational watching the group dynamics. Everyone in the class knows that everyone else in the group is struggling to conceive a child. Although sad for themselves, by and large they are happy to hear when other women in the class get pregnant. They all seem to be rooting for each other because it gives them hope for themselves. Yet, if they know of a friend outside the circle who has not struggled to get pregnant, it is much more difficult to be happy for them. Somehow it seems easier to feel compassion for someone when you know they have suffered a bit or feel your same pain. Each of us can probably point to a friend or two who have had an easy time of conceiving and having a child. Now they seem to "have it all" or at least have exactly what you want. In fact, they may seem downright insensitive about your fertility woes.

You want a child, you've worked hard for one, yet your dream is not yet realized. This can lead to feelings of resentment, anger, and even hatred toward your friends, which can be a very unpleasant feeling. In some instances, we are simply projecting our needs and frustrations onto them. The enemy is in you and you are in her. Your friends or family may be a symbol of the desires you have been denied. Recognize that they represent what your life would be like if you had children. It is not they who are making you feel bitter and angry it is you who are doing that. If you are isolating yourself from your friends, that is your choice. Again, people will never control what they say or how they say it, but you can control how you react to it.

Remember the psychologist who once said that if you put 100 people in a room and were told you could exchange problems with one of them; you would probably never do it? As the Buddhists say, "all life is suffering." This is a basic and noble truth. It's the story of the woman trying to find the mustard seed from the one house that does not know suffering; she never finds it. Everybody has something that makes them unhappy or something that creates a source of irritation in their life. If they don't have that something, it's because they have learned to adapt, adjust, and "acclimatize" to their environment. This results in a change in attitude which ultimately helps them better cope with their problems.

If all of your friends are getting pregnant and you feel pain and resentment, rest assured that they have other issues they are dealing with that bring pain into their lives. It may be well hidden from you, but you must trust that it is there. Yoga teaches us that since suffering is a basic premise of life, we need to show compassion for everyone, even our enemies. One technique that we find particularly useful when feeling challenged by not having something you want in life, is to look at someone who has less or even more challenges. By doing this you will begin to feel grateful for what you do have. Have you ever watched the evening news or picked up a copy of *People* magazine and seen real-life stories of suffering and pain that are far greater than your own? When you hit a rough spot in your life, think about expressing gratitude because, believe it or not, there is a gift or lesson waiting for you on the other side.

If your cousin had an immaculate conception at the age of 46, your sister has eight children, and your best friend keeps having little "oopsies," recognize these words of wisdom your mother told you when you were little: *life is not fair*. Although there is generally nothing we can do about it, accepting the fact that life is unfair goes a long way in ridding the anxiety of infertility. In fact, accepting the fact that life is unfair can go a long way in ridding any anxiety in life.

Practice giving up the feelings of jealousy you might have toward your friends and start giving more compassion and love. As the karmic wheel of life continues to spin, you will see that what you sow is indeed what you reap. By planting seeds of jealousy, more jealousy will grow. By planting seeds of compassion, more compassion will be shown to you. Then, one day, quite without realizing it, you will see that you have risen above it all. You will be happy for your friends' happiness because you will also be able to see their suffering. In the end, evaluating whether someone else's pain is greater or less than yours is nothing more than a judgment call.

WEEK 6 ACTIVITY 3: REDUCING THE JEALOUSY STRESSOR

Create an altar of gratitude. Take five votive candles and line them up on a table or flat surface. On a sheet of paper, write down five things for which you are truly grateful. Look at them, meditate upon them, and allow the feeling of gratitude to permeate your entire being. Then, out loud, say the first thing for which you are grateful. Light the first votive candle and then say aloud, "I am thankful for _____ because _____". Look at your paper and say the second thing on your gratitude list. Light the second candle. Repeat the phrase, "I am thankful for _____ because _____". Proceed with the third, fourth, and fifth candle in the same way. When all candles are lit, spend a few more minutes in silence, holding the feeling of gratitude in your heart. When you are finished, blow out your candles but keep the paper with your list on it. Hang this list on your refrigerator, in your bathroom, or in another place that will be a daily reminder of those things for which you are thankful.

"I'm Not Worthy" Stressor

This particular stressor can manifest itself in two different ways. The first is through our inability to recognize or accept gifts from others and the second is our belief that we are not worthy because of something we said or did in the past. Let's first discuss the idea that we are not able to truly accept gifts from others.

There was a woman in one of our classes who was having a beastly time trying to get pregnant. She expressed anxiety over seeing a member of her family who always put on the puppy dog eyes, grabbed her hand, and said, "I just know you will have a baby one day. Try to stay optimistic." This student said she never knew how to respond and that every time she saw this family member she was overcome by stress and agitation. This stressor could be easily eliminated if we better learned how to graciously accept gifts from others. You would never turn away a gift that someone wrapped for you in pretty paper and tied with a bow. Why do we turn away the non-tangible gifts we are given every day? If someone is rooting for you to get pregnant, open your heart enough to accept the gift and thank them. If they "just know you will get pregnant one day" then say, "I really appreciate the gift of your kind words and good wishes." Even if you sense they don't really mean it, take the gift anyway because good energy follows good intentions (have we hit you over the head enough with that saying yet?).

The second aspect of the "I'm not worthy" stressor is thinking that there is something innately unworthy about us. Maybe we terminated a pregnancy when we were younger, maybe we have doubt as to our own ability to truly be a parent, or maybe we wonder if this is really the kind of world into which we ought to bring another life. The ghosts of the past want to live again. No matter how much therapy we have done or how much we intellectually know our thinking is flawed, it is difficult to change our belief patterns. Fertility will truly be enhanced, however, when we stop focusing on our unworthiness and begin to focus on our worthiness; when we stop giving all our power to other people and to our past experiences. Be worthy, feel worthy. Know that you are one of God's highest creatures and that if you cannot imagine it, you cannot create it. Walt Disney once said, "If you can dream it, you can achieve it." Begin your dream!

Love your body, love yourself, and accept the gifts the world has to offer you. The more you are willing to receive, the more the universe will give you and the more you will have to give to others. Be kind to yourself and open your heart to all of your beauty and simultaneously, all of your faults. The healing process begins with you.

Close your eyes and inhale through your nose. At the top of the inhale when your lungs and diaphragm feel completely filled with air, suspend your breath and say the following affirmation to yourself three times:

I am happy

I am healthy

I am holy

Now exhale out all of the air and say the affirmation out loud three times:

I am happy

I am healthy

I am holy

Repeat this mantra practice for at least five minutes. Remember the reason we do these exercises is to change the way we are thinking at a subconscious level and to bring greater peace and happiness into our lives. The process is not meant to stress you or make you pass out. If you feel any tension in your breathing patterns whatsoever, adjust the number of times you say the mantra to more closely complement the rhythm of your own breathing.

Ego Stressors

Along the lines of the letting-go muscle, trying to conceive can be stressful because we wish to control all aspects of the process. We are taught as children that if we work hard enough in life we can achieve anything our hearts desire. In most cases, this is true but not in the world of fertility. How is it possible that we have changed our diet, given up caffeine, have sex every other night, stand on our heads after intercourse, read books on conception, and still do not have a baby? There is not one more thing we could possibly do. For those of us who are "type A personalities," losing control of this situation is quite unpleasant. It begins to shake the very foundation of who we are. If I am not to be a mother, then who or what am I to be? Questions like these can lead to a loss of self-esteem and even spiritual crisis. We begin to ask existential questions like, "Why me?" or "How come I am being punished?" This is where we really need to understand the nature of our ego.

Our egos are always looking for something upon which they can attach. It is our egos that define us as banker, wife, mother, sister, athlete, rich, poor, Catholic, Jewish, American, fat, skinny, or otherwise. We want to be special; to have a label or mark by which we can identify ourselves. Now there's nothing wrong with that. Everyone has certain ego identifications, which are completely normal. Unfortunately, we get trapped into thinking we are our egos and sometimes our ego identification is negative rather than positive. This is where we can get into trouble. Think about the woman in the newspaper who is in a physically abusive relationship. Despite numerous beatings, she never leaves the situation.

My Ego

Well, how did you do on Activity 5? How did you describe yourself? In his book, The Power of Now, *Eckhart Tolle points out that most of us define ourselves by the following:*

- *My possessions*
- *My job*
- *My social status*
- *My recognitions*
- *My knowledge*
- *My education*
- *My physical appearance*
- *My special abilities*

- *My relationships*
- *My personal or family history*
- *My belief system*
- *My politics*
- *My nationalism*
- *My race*
- *My religion*

Why? She never leaves because her ego identification is that of being "the abused." It is her label. Her ego is too vested and too attached to change her situation. The mind prefers to attach itself to that which is known and familiar rather than to move forward toward that which is unfamiliar or new. The unknown is dangerous to the mind because it has no control over it.

One of the students in Tami's Tools for Healing class who had experienced a miscarriage at 20 weeks of pregnancy approached her after class regarding a discussion the class had on ego identification. "I realize for the first time," she said, "that my ego identification has been that of a miscarriage victim. My actions, my feelings, my thinking, and my sadness are all created around this ego identification of loss." Recognizing her own, innate patterns helped the student detach from this idea of loss and move toward greater healing. She was now able to see the ego label affixed to her and how that label was no longer useful. For this particular student, detaching from the label was the beginning of putting closure to her loss. That is the power of ego self-study; when you have an "A-ha moment" it can be very profound, even life-altering.

Quick Yoga Tip

"When you have a negative thought, instantly replace it with a positive thought."
Yoga Sutras of Patanjali

WEEK 6 ACTIVITY 5: UNDERSTANDING YOUR EGO

Please complete this simple exercise. With a piece of paper and pen, imagine that you have a pen pal you have never met who lives in another country. Who are you? Tell him or her every little thing about yourself. Do the exercise now.

This exercise is designed to help you recognize your ego tendencies so that you might more clearly understand that you are in all things and all things are in you. They say the eyes of a person are the windows to their soul. Sit opposite your partner or a friend and gaze into their eyes. If you prefer to do this alone, find a mirror and stare into it. The gazing should be broken into three sections that are three minutes each in length. For the first three minutes, while gazing into your partner's eyes, let the focus of your meditation be on yourself. Let all your awareness be centered around the idea of who you are in the eyes of your partner.

For the next three minutes, let the focus of your attention be on your partner or the person in the mirror. Notice how their face changes or how the candle flickers and what their eyes might be telling you. For the last three minutes, focus on the world around you, including the space and energy not occupied by people or things. It is helpful if you have a third person timing the sessions for you, otherwise if you do it alone, you are likely to break your concentration. Remember that while you are focusing on yourself, your partner is focusing on himself. When you are focusing on "other," you are focusing on him and he is focusing on you. You can call the three segments "self," "other," and "surroundings."

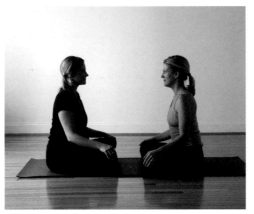

Gazing (Trataka)

Job Stressors

So many women who are trying to conceive wonder if quitting their jobs would reduce their stress and, therefore, enhance their chances of getting pregnant. This is a very difficult decision and one that needs careful contemplation. Here's the problem. So much of what we do for a living shapes our ego identity. You may think that quitting your job will relieve your stress but you might find it even more stressful to be without an identifying label. If you quit your job and don't get pregnant right away, do you know what you will do? Many women find that they are more miserable once they leave their jobs because they become bored, feel as though they are not contributing, or lose a sense of self-worth. Remember, too, that if you quit your job to focus on conceiving a child then your stress emphasis will be on conception. Your chances of feeling more stressed out about fertility will likely be magnified. Granted you won't feel tension over your job anymore, but you will likely find something else to worry about. In addition, financial strains may be more stressful than the job ever was.

So, what's the solution to this dilemma? The first step is to determine why you want to quit. In determining this answer, please ask yourself the following questions and then study your answers to gain greater insight into your career stressors.

- Do you like your current job? What makes it good or bad?
- Do you like being in this particular industry or would you change it if you could?
- Do you need to work for financial purposes?
- What would you do with your time if you didn't have this job?
- Does the stress of your job interfere with your overall happiness?
- Have you always dreamed of doing this type of work?
- Are you well compensated for your work?
- Do you get the "Sunday blues?"
- If time, money, and energy were not an issue, what would you do?

If the sum total of your responses actually does add up to needing a change in your career, we suggest you employ the help of a certified life coach. At PDtM we have a life coach on staff who regularly meets with women to discuss these very challenges. In working with a life coach you not only address your dissatisfactions with the current state of affairs, you engage in activities that help you devise a plan and seek potential options that most harmoniously fit with your life goals.

Delay of Gratification Stressor

"I want the world. I want the whole world. I want to lock it all up in my pocket. It's my bar of chocolate. Give it to me now ... I want it now, Daddy."

VERUCA SALT IN WILLY WONKA AND THE CHOCOLATE FACTORY

Infertility is stressful because it is an exercise in delay of gratification in a very fast-paced and immediate society. It's like wanting a Barbie when you're six years old but being told by your mom that you can't have one until you're 16. Or, going to 20 different baby showers and being the only one who always leaves without the baby. At some point it's just considered a cruel and unusual punishment.

It's hard enough knowing that you will have to wait at least nine months for the arrival of your baby. If you are having difficulty conceiving, then every time you get your period or have an unsuccessful cycle you may feel a bit anxious or disappointed. You may find yourself wishing you could press the fast-forward button just to see how the story ends.

There is a great concept in yoga called *"rta."* Rta, in a sense, is the flow of the universe. It's the idea that everything has a right time, a right place, and a right way in which to manifest. Everything in the universe is in complete equilibrium and exists in a duality. For every day, night must follow. We have a left hand and a right hand, a left eye and a right eye. There is the sun and the moon, man and woman, young and old, hot and cold, birth and death. In order to truly understand what cold is, we have to first experience hot. To appreciate a rainbow, we have to know what a storm feels like. This is to say that all experiences are relative based on your frame of reference. In order for one thing to exist, its exact opposite must also exist. That means that for every hardship, the seeds of opportunity must also be present.

In his book, *When Bad Things Happen to Good People*, Harold Kushner likens a tapestry to the trials and tribulations of daily life. On one side of the tapestry all the threads look disorganized. There are many colors, different lengths, and some threads even look like they are tangled with other threads. When you turn the tapestry over, however, it makes a perfectly glorious masterpiece. This is a great metaphor for understanding the rta. You may feel at times like you got the "short thread" so to speak, but after looking more closely you may see that your short thread was necessary to make a more beautiful tapestry.

So many women who come through our doors at PDtM say the same thing: going through infertility has been incredibly difficult, but looking back, they would never change the experience because they have gained and grown so much through the process:

Neither PDtM would exist nor would this book be written if Tami and Beth had not each experienced infertility and loss. Go back to the idea that every challenge in life is also a gift in disguise. What you will learn about yourself, the world and other people will be invaluable gifts at some point in your life. Maybe it will just give you a greater appreciation for life and the gift of the child once he or she does enter into your life. Again, be open to receiving the gifts the world has to give you. You may be very impatient to have everything now, Veruca Salt, but trust that there is an order and a pattern for your life. You can swim with the tides of existence or swim against them and feel very frustrated, out of control and unhappy in the process. Trust that everything is as it should be in this very moment.

WEEK 6 ACTIVITY 8: SOFTENING THE DELAY OF GRATIFICATION STRESSOR

Do the "Make a Gift" activity in the box on p. 165. This is your opportunity to express your vision for motherhood through the creative process. Creating a work of art, or writing, takes time and discipline. Everything that we envision or think about in our minds must somehow make its way from a subtle thought into matter. Once again, you have to envision it if you are to create it, but the creativity process takes time. Not only will this exercise illustrate the importance of patience and delay of gratification, it also stimulates our creative center located in the second chakra. Fittingly, the second chakra not only governs our creativity but also our reproductive organs and system, appetite, feelings, food, and sex.

Burn Out Stressor

If you are already going through infertility treatment then we cannot dismiss "burn out" as a cause of stress. Going to see the doctor, ultrasounds, taking meds, having procedures, the two-week wait, the disappointment; the cycle seems unending. In fact, you don't even like sex anymore. Having a baby has gotten to be one big pain in the backside, literally, with all those injections. So what choices do you really have? Do you really want to stop?

Burn out happens when a stressful situation is ongoing. You may begin to feel like you do not have the resources necessary to adequately cope with your desire to have a child. You may feel the same physical symptoms of stress, but burn out includes an emotional exhaustion and an increasingly negative attitude toward your life situation. People with high expectations for themselves are most likely to "burn out." Their compulsive desire to achieve a goal can become an obsession with detrimental effects. Unrealistic goals are set and they erroneously believe that anything is possible with the right amount of work or effort. When they take on more than they can handle they cannot maintain that intensity over a sustained period of time and burn out results. Fertility burn out can occur when the desire to conceive becomes an obsession that occupies your every thought and affects your ability to be happy, think clearly or plan your future. You may find yourself saying, "I can't do this anymore," yet you continue to do it.

When we see this type of worn-out behavior at PDtM, we often encourage patients to take a break. It often requires more courage to stop than to keep going with "baby-making sex" or fertility treatment because most patients want to stay on the treadmill. Unlearning a patterned behavior can be as difficult as learning it in the first place. We have all heard stories about couples who "stopped trying" or adopted, only to find that they got pregnant shortly thereafter. Unfortunately, there is no scientific evidence that "giving up" promotes pregnancy. From a yoga perspective, stopping for a while can have dramatic effects on our energetic well-being. Changing your focus can help you recharge your batteries and assist with making difficult decisions a lot easier. Have you ever had a tough day that you thought was insurmountable only to feel refreshed and better armed to tackle your problems after a good night's rest? This is one example of how momentum can change by taking a break.

Make a Gift

Begin thinking about the child you are meant to have and choose one of the exercises below to give to the child as a gift one day. Work on your project over the remaining seven weeks of this book. Place the gift to this child in your "hope chest" or time capsule until such a time when it is suitable to give it to him/her directly.

- *A cross stitch or needlepoint*
- *Paint-by-number picture or free-hand drawing*
- *A letter expressing how much you have anticipated the child's arrival*
- *A poem or song*

WEEK 6 ACTIVITY 9: SOFTENING THE BURN OUT STRESSOR

The best cure for burn out is to stop or reduce the activity causing burn out and begin to focus on (emphasize) something that you truly love. Make a pact with yourself here and now to find time to do the things you love, if only for one hour, three times a week. Don't wait for "quiet time" to find you because it just won't. Rest and relaxation are seldom available; you have to reach out and grab them by the tail. Make a plan to do three things for yourself this week that you wouldn't ordinarily find time to do. They don't have to be lofty aspirations.

How about taking a walk in nature, or calling an old friend for a cup of tea? Maybe stop by church and light a candle and just pray for 20 minutes? How about making an appointment at the spa for a relaxation massage or buying an erotic massage oil to use on your spouse or partner? Change it up! Surprise yourself but, most importantly, commit to finding this time. Not only will your burn out be doused but you will also begin to take the emphasis off your obsessive behavior and focus, more thoroughly, on something truly positive for your mind and spirit. So, remember, you are in charge of your pace and fertility, even though you're not ultimately in control.

WEEK 6 ACTIVITY 10: THE CURE-ALL PRACTICE: BREATH OF DE-STRESS

Inhale, hold the breath for a second and then exhale while counting 1....2....3. Start by counting quickly at first, even at lightning speed if you need to. Do this a few more times. Now inhale slowly, hold the breath for five seconds and then exhale while counting slowly 1....2....3....4....5.... Do this again. This time inhale, hold the breath for 8 seconds and then exhale very slowly while mentally counting 1....2....3....4....5....6....7....8. With each round, keep elongating the count and therefore the length of your exhale. As your exhales begin to lengthen your inhales will naturally lengthen on their own.

What We've Learned

As mentioned earlier, stress is that upon which we place emphasis. By its very definition then, stress is an internal factor. The external event does not cause the stress, our internal reactions, attitudes, and thoughts do. Unless we are suffering from physical pain, stress is a mental function which produces physical symptoms. By getting "out of our heads" or quieting the mind, we can greatly impact our ability to handle stress.

If you are not used to controlling your thought process in this way, you may find the "quieting" exercises in this chapter frustrating because the mind does not like to be still. This is particularly true during times of anxiety or restlessness. If you practice these techniques during times of low stress when the mind is more still, you will have greater success in using them during high stress times when the mind is noisy and much more difficult to control.

Letting Go of Attachment and Disappointment

SOME OF YOU who are reading this book may have already experienced sadness, loss, or disappointment in your desire to have a child. Perhaps you have not achieved pregnancy after trying for a long time. Maybe you have miscarried, had a stillbirth, or experienced multiple rounds of failed fertility cycles. Feelings of loss are also common. It could be loss of a child, a dream, money, time, certain relationships, or even loss of your familiar self. These experiences can be more than just frustrating; they can be devastating and life-altering.

Within your conception tool box, you will need different ways to help cope with the feelings of disappointment and loss that may accompany your fertility journey. We would like to provide you with two different sets of tools. The first grouping is for when you are in crisis mode and really need a quick fix. It may not repair the whole infrastructure, but it will keep your house in good working order. The second set of tools is offered from the yoga tradition. The ancient yogis had some really interesting advice on how to deal with disappointment that may require a lot more soul searching and reflection. Although a bit more esoteric in nature, the second set of tools will work on the foundation of your house and ensure it is built on solid ground.

Dealing with Disappointment: Crisis Mode Tools

SEEK SUPPORT

Spouse, family, and friends are a good place to start but you may find you are consoling them just as much as they are consoling you. As mentioned in the beginning of this section, most women do not go beyond family and friends for support because they are discouraged by cost or don't know who to call. There are plenty of places to get referrals, including your local fertility clinics, which may even offer free psychological support for their patients.

Research has also shown that women who seek support during fertility treatment have higher conception rates. Try seeking guidance from a holistic practitioner, psychotherapist, or local fertility support group such as Resolve or the American Fertility Association (AFA). With online communities growing in number, finding someone to "chat" with who may have had similar loss or disappointment is also an option in helping you heal.

NURTURE YOURSELF

Become your own bowl of chicken soup by unplugging for a day of self-healing. Take a day off work, book a massage, get an acupuncture treatment, have tea with a friend, or lay on the couch with a good book. Do the things you love for one day, without guilt and without apology.

FEED THE SPIRIT

Many women who have experienced loss or disappointment are also in a state of spiritual crisis. They wonder why this is happening to them or question what the "master plan" really is all about. They may find talking with a member of their church, temple, or synagogue is really therapeutic. Stopping by their place of worship, lighting a candle, creating a ritual, or turning to prayer can also be helpful.

TAKE A WALK

Engaging the senses by walking in nature can change the momentum of your day. In addition to being a "fertility-friendly" exercise, walking also provides quiet time for you to spend with your thoughts. Take long, deep breaths and engage the senses while you do it. Notice the sounds you hear, the smells in the air and the way a leaf or flower might feel to the touch. As you walk and breathe deeply, imagine you are taking in positive energy and getting rid of the negative.

FIND INSPIRATION

When you are feeling particularly vulnerable by loss or disappointment, it can be very helpful finding inspiration from other people who have also experienced difficulty. Read biographies, attend lectures, listen to audio tapes, or spend time researching to gain a better understanding of how other people may have survived their challenging times.

LEARN TO MEDITATE

Meditation allows us to see our emotions as they come and go. The more we practice this ancient technique, the more we are able to step outside of our mind and body and find more lasting peace in times of crisis, loss, or disappointment (see Chapter 11 for more details).

EXPRESS GRATITUDE

Some women find it helpful to create an altar of thanksgiving. Try the ritual of gratitude that was provided for you in an earlier section of this book.

Take five votive candles and line them up on a table or flat surface. On a sheet of paper, write down five things for which you are truly grateful. Look at them, meditate upon them, and allow the feeling of gratitude to permeate your entire being. Then, out loud, say the first thing for which you are grateful. Light the first votive candle and then say aloud, "I am thankful for _____ because _____. Look at your paper and say the second thing on your gratitude list. Light the second candle. Repeat the phrase, "I am thankful for _____ because _____. Proceed with the third, fourth, and fifth candle in the same way. When all candles are lit, spend a few more minutes in silence, meditating. When you are finished, blow out your candles but keep the paper with your list on it. Hang this list on your refrigerator, in your bathroom, or in another location that will be a daily reminder of those things for which you are thankful.

SERVE SOMEONE ELSE

When you are feeling challenged by life, try walking a mile in another person's shoes. Find a soul that needs help and happily serve them. There are limitless numbers of ways you can approach this project so think about a way to serve that will be most meaningful for both you and the recipient of your gift. Here are some ideas: serve at a soup kitchen, help someone move, mow the lawn for your elderly neighbor, make cookies for a friend who has been feeling blue, fill boxes with clothes you no longer wear and take them to a women's shelter or volunteer at a local orphanage.

You will find that by stepping outside of yourself and focusing energy on another human being, your own pain will lessen. You may find that the person you are serving ends up really serving you.

Dealing with Disappointment: Long-Term Strategy

Before we discuss the more esoteric ways of dealing with disappointment, it is important for all of us to acknowledge that feeling a sense of loss or being stuck is completely normal during this time because the desire for a child is, perhaps, one of our most primal instincts. All species have the desire to procreate, to mother, to have offspring, to proliferate their species; humans are no different. It is completely natural to feel disappointed when this seemingly natural process begins to feel unnatural or forced.

That being said, the yoga tradition states that we tend to get ourselves into trouble because we create problems and then don't fully know how to free ourselves from them. One of the biggest ways we do this is through our desires. In both the yoga philosophy and

Buddhism it is thought that human suffering is caused by our attachments and desires. Even desire for the most noble of things like having children or enlightenment, for instance, leads to suffering because if the seeker does not find what he or she is looking for, he or she will be unhappy or feel unfulfilled. The trick, they say, is to eliminate the desire entirely. If there is no desire, there can be no pain, no disappointment, no sadness, etc. This, of course, is much easier said than done, particularly when we are talking about ridding a desire as sacred as life itself, that of procreation and having a child.

We do not claim to be experts in the esoteric meaning of these sacred teachings, but we don't believe the Buddha or the ancient yogis meant that we should walk through life like zombies feeling indifferent and apathetic. Perhaps these sages meant that it is helpful to approach life's desires with a bit of detachment from the outcome in order to live a happier, less stress-filled existence.

Exercising detachment means that you understand, at a deep level, that you will never be completely fulfilled by the fruits of your desires. You are able to look upon your desires from a more global perspective and understand that just as fulfillment of your desires will never complete you, unfulfillment will never truly defeat you. You can see your desires, but do not feel attached to them.

The Cycle of Desire

Think about how desire might manifest itself in your life by contemplating this scenario. You work really hard and save money because you want to buy a shiny red convertible. After you drive out of the showroom you start to think about how great it would be to take a road trip to show off your new car. While you are driving to your four-star resort, a place where you've always wanted to stay, you realize that you will need a bigger garage to keep your car safe. You've wanted to buy a house anyway because your current apartment is really small. You tell yourself that when you buy your house you're going to make sure it has a big backyard too, because you love gardening. You work harder, save more money, buy the house and then feel perhaps the rooms should be filled with babies because it is too big and lonely for just you and your husband. It is time to share your life and your knowledge with a child. After you have the child you experience sleepless nights and long for a full eight hours of rest. Then you want to quit your job and spend more time with your child because you are just too stressed out. The story could go on and on.

You see, all of us have desires. The trouble is, our desires are never-ending. Even when we achieve them, more desires suddenly present themselves. Today you want a child; tomorrow you will want something else, symbolically. Don't fool yourself into thinking that your life will be fulfilled, complete, or eternally happy once you have a child because it won't. You will likely feel incredibly blessed, you may feel that you have found your life's calling, but don't underestimate the power of your innate, incessant, and so-very-human desires. The bottom line is this: all of us just want to be happy; thinking that the car, the house, the vacation, or the baby is going to bring it to us is completely erroneous.

Tools for Coping with Disappointment

So if we follow this line of thinking and buy into the idea that yearning leads to suffering, what are some tools for coping with the desire and the disappointment that accompany it? Again, we turn to the ancient text of the *Yoga Sutras of Patanjali*. There are five obstacles in life that feed our cravings and ultimately lead to pain and disappointment. These five obstacles are called *"kleshas"* or afflictions and they are delusion, sense of ego, attachment, rejection and fear. It is the goal in life to identify, uproot, and unwind these habitual patterns.

AVIDYA: MIS-KNOWING/DELUSION

The first of these afflictions is avidya, which is delusion or mis-knowing, and it is believed to be a root cause of our suffering. It is different from ignorance because ignorance implies a certain amount of stupidity. Avidya is more unconscious. Now, consider this in terms of your own fertility. If you have experienced a lot of loss, you may incorrectly believe that the loss will never leave you or that it will happen again. It becomes a part of you and embeds itself into your psyche. You feel defeated and unable to move forward with any additional fertility treatments or options. This is avidya because you are "mis-knowing" the truth about your fertility. You might experience further loss or you might not. The truth is, if you don't try to have a child you most certainly never will.

The feelings of loss do not hold onto you, you hold onto them. If you honor them and then let them go, you free yourself. This is not to say that we forget about the child we carried and lost. It *is* to say we honor the child by holding a place in our heart for its spirit but learn to let go of the negative feelings surrounding the event. By doing this, we do not let our negative experience cloud our perception or judgment for the future.

ASMITA: SENSE OF EGO

Asmita is simply your sense of self or ego. In the previous chapter we talked about how your sense of *I-ness* during the fertility process can be a big stressor. Asmita expresses itself with statements like the following: "Nobody suffers like me" or, "I should be getting more attention from my doctor." How about, "I know I'm right" or, "I deserve to get pregnant." Life is all about us; our pain, our sorrow, our joy, and our heartache. When we don't get what we think we deserve we experience sorrow and disappointment.

This is where compassion can be extremely healing. In order to overcome the klesha of Asmita you need to go outside of yourself and begin to see that all people experience some form of pain or suffering. Think about ways in which you can serve others to overcome the ego pain you feel yourself. Visit a children's cancer home, feed an elderly person, or volunteer at a soup kitchen. If you think your doctor should be paying more attention to you, put yourself in their shoes and think about the hundreds of other patients who also demand their attention. Leave the house of your mind and its emotional nature to experience the ego nature of another human being.

RAGAS: ATTACHMENT

We are all very familiar with ragas. It is the affliction of attachment, of wanting things we don't have, not appreciating what we do have or wanting more of it. We like to call it the klesha of possessions and obsessions. Each of us can probably think of something to which we feel attached. Perhaps it's that shoulder-padded jacket from 1992 that takes up space in your closet but with which you have not been able to part. Maybe you are attached to certain ideas about your fertility, like how a child will come to you or what medical or holistic procedures you will or will not do. Perhaps you are attached to a particular physician even though you may have lost faith in his or her methods or medical advice. You really have to become mindful of your attachments and ask yourself if they serve you or not on this conception journey. You may find that most of your attachments are rather benign and may not lead to a whole lot of sorrow or pain, but some can become very rigid beliefs or even physical or mental addictions. Addictions can affect our health, quality of life, our ability to conceive, and the overall well-being of our offspring.

We all know a story about a professional athlete who becomes attached to steroids because he believes it will enhance his performance on the field, or the alcoholic who drowns her sorrows in martinis every night. How about the runner who can't miss a day at the gym or the stressed-out businessperson who is never separated from his or her cell phone and mobile email device? Addictions to caffeine, drugs, sex, food, smoking, exercise, and even technology are attachments of avidya (mis-knowing). We falsely believe that we can't give them up, we need them or think that our happiness or well-being is somehow dependent upon them. If we needed it yesterday, we must need it today and we are going to require it tomorrow. Letting go of our attachments and addictions, be they good ones or bad, ultimately leads to freedom.

Tackling Addiction

Within Oriental Medicine (OM), there is no standard approach to tackling any addiction. Everyone is different; their reasons and motivations for using are different. Their responses to using are different. And their responses to quitting are different. For this reason, it is best to consult a trained practitioner of OM.

Smoking and Infertility

The negative effect that smoking cigarettes has on fertility is well documented. Research shows that smoking in women speeds the aging process, increases the likelihood of genetic abnormalities in eggs, hastens menopause, increases likelihood of miscarriage, and decreases the effectiveness of ovarian stimulation during ART. If you smoke, quitting is the single best thing you can do to improve fertility. There are many avenues to help people quit smoking. These include medication, nicotine patches, nicotine gum, support groups, hypnotherapy, individual counseling, acupuncture and herbal therapy and probably many others. Whatever method works will be fine. However, if you can do it, it is probably best to quit without the use of drugs or nicotine. But, if these interventions prove necessary, it is still much better than continuing with this habit which can negatively impact your fertility.

In general, addictive behaviors tend to be motivated by an inner anxiety. For whatever mal-adaptive reasons, people find comfort and calm from smoking. Accordingly, acupuncture and herbal treatments will almost always treat the mind and the spirit as well as the body. In the short term, these interventions can moderate the symptoms of withdrawal. These include, but are not limited to: irritability, anxiety, nervousness, headaches, insomnia, digestive disturbances (including elimination), cough, sore throat, and fatigue. In addition, acupuncture has been shown to be very effective in curbing cravings. This effect works not only on nicotine, but also heroin, cocaine, alcohol, chocolate, over-eating, and anything for which one may develop a pathological desire.

This is how OM can help people deal with the acute phase of addiction. We must also address the underlying motivator or cause of the addiction. In OM, the Heart is the mansion of the spirit as mentioned in Chapter 2. So by strengthening the Heart we can help to contain, or calm, the spirit. This reduces the need that some feel for nicotine to "calm and comfort." A calmer spirit will have less need for mind-altering chemicals. OM can also improve circulation to, and healing of, the lungs. It can promote the body's ability to detoxify and eliminate the chemicals introduced by the smoke.

While OM treatments are individualized, there are dietary and lifestyle recommendations that would be helpful for most people who are trying to quit. For one, avoid situations that you associate with smoking. For example, if you always go outside the building during the breaks, stop going outside. Once you are on more solid footing, you may be better able to withstand temptation. But early on, you need to make this easy on yourself whenever possible. Some people use lollipops, but we recommend that you carry a toothbrush and toothpaste. Whenever you want to have a cigarette, brush your teeth. This will help satisfy the hand-mouth connection, as well as freshen your breath. You should also breathe deeply. One of the reasons that smoking may seem to calm is because it forces us to take deep breaths. This has a more calming effect than the smoke. Nicotine is actually a stimulant. You may also want to write a list of reasons why you want/need to quit, which will probably include the many benefits quitting will have on your fertility. Consult this list when confronted with cravings. You may want to seek help from the others around you to support your decision to quit smoking.

OM can help you quit. If you are ready, it can make the process a lot easier and increase your chances for pregnancy. If you are not ready, it will help you get ready. If you need more help finding motivation please consult the American Lung Association. They can be found at www.lungusa.org or call 1-800-LUNGUSA.

Beth writes:

I was a closet smoker in graduate school, nervously puffing on a butt whenever a big deadline or paper was due. Once I started practicing yoga, my desire for a smoke was one of my first bad habits to go. As we mentioned above, it's hypothesized that smokers find the practice of smoking relaxing because it makes them take deep, mindful inhales. As yoga taught me to do the same, I found I got the same calming results without the tar and nicotine—and with an added dose of prana.

DVESA: AVERSIONS

Dvesa is the opposite of ragas (attachment). It is our aversions or dislikes. In this case we find ourselves staying away from people, things, situations, or thoughts that we think will cause us pain. If they caused us pain in the past, then we avoid them or begin to hate them for fear these things will cause us pain in the future. As we all know, hatred is an incredibly powerful emotion that often moves us in directions of negative speaking, thinking or acting.

Let's say you go skiing once and break your leg. It is reasonable to think you might grow to hate skiing and may even avoid going for the rest of your life. The healing and happiness comes when you begin to evaluate the situations which caused the broken leg. Did you attempt a hill that was way beyond your skill level? Did your friends force you into jumping an icy mogul? Did you wipe out and break your leg because you were showing off? Was it just a fluke accident? Once you ask the question "why," begin to think about how your actions or your thinking might have contributed to the broken leg. Now ask what you can do to avoid hurting yourself in the future. Next time, perhaps you stick to the bunny hill or enroll in ski school. Maybe you avoid the moguls or swallow your pride and let everybody else be the "hot dog." Clarity often comes by delving into the specific avidya that caused the aversion in the first place. At the end of the day you may choose to just sip hot chocolate in the ski chalet while everybody else enjoys the slopes but, after having thought about why it is you avoid skiing, you may find new courage to do it again. What happens if you do it again and love it? Now you've changed your entire perspective of skiing or at least softened the hatred you feel toward it.

If you are having difficulty getting pregnant, the solution may not be as easy as sipping a hot toddy by a warm fire, particularly if you are thinking, "I hate the medicine," "I hate my doctor," "I hate IVF," "I hate my husband right now," "I hate the two-week wait." Ask yourself why you feel hatred or have an aversion to these things and see if, by exploring the reasons or finding different solutions, you can soften your grumpy personality or gain the courage to face these aversions head on. You just might find the clarity you need to turn your hatred into tolerance or acceptance.

You may have heard that love is the closest emotion to hate. We would like to present the idea that hope is the flip side of hate. For everything that you hate or fear, you also have an innate hope that the same things will bring you happiness. For example, you might fear IVF, but also hope that it gets you pregnant. You might hate your husband right now, but you also hope that he will be more compassionate to your situation. It is important to develop steadiness in your thinking and in your emotions. Mental steadiness means that when fear and hate arise, we don't ride the emotional roller coaster with them. We keep balanced in our approach and realize that the ups and downs, the hope and fears, the love and hatred are all a part of life and cannot destroy our ability to be happy.

ABHINIVESA: FEAR

The fifth and final klesha is fear, an emotion most of us experience quite often in our lives. It comes in all shapes and sizes. There is fear of failure, fear of being wrong, fear of getting hurt, fear of change, fear of growing old, fear of regret, fear of loss, and fear of death, to name just a few. Understanding your fears is a critical part of moving beyond loss and disappointment because fear can paralyze you. Think about how many times fear has driven you to take a certain action or not to take action. We are not suggesting that you go out and find courage in the face of life-threatening events. Petting a stranger's pit bull to overcome your fear of dogs is not a good idea. We are suggesting that you take a closer look at those things that scare you and ask yourself if your fear is preventing you from being happy. If so, how can you take action to help rid or soften your feelings of fear?

Noelle was a student at PDtM who had suffered three miscarriages, some as late as 22 weeks of pregnancy. For her, the problem was not getting pregnant, it was staying pregnant. Two of her pregnancies had happened spontaneously and the third was the result of IVF. She was traumatized by her loss and felt a deep sense of fear about moving forward with another IVF and genetic testing only to have her hopes shattered by miscarriage. Noelle knew she had to make a decision about whether or not to proceed with treatment but she was paralyzed by her fear of miscarriage. She did not feel that she could endure another pregnancy only to have her dreams of having a child shattered by another loss. Noelle decided to delay her decision and focus on getting her body and mind in the best possible shape to carry a child. She started by getting acupuncture every week and having a nutritionist evaluate her diet. She also needed some tools for stress management as she had recently changed jobs and was spending more and more time in the office and less time relaxing and doing the things she truly loved. She joined a yoga class and learned various breathing techniques and visualizations to help induce relaxation. It took a lot of courage, but Noelle also decided to see a sex therapist because she realized the losses and her corresponding mood swings were causing a strain in her marriage. Not so much sexually, but she felt the intimacy they had shared had dissipated since the miscarriages. Noelle felt the "best friend" she had married was no longer there for her. His way of coping was very different from hers and it created a sense of separation between them. At first she started seeing the therapist by herself and then later asked her husband to join her. Noelle spent the better part of four months working on getting herself and her marriage "back in shape."

At the end of this time, Noelle realized that she had gained a new sense of confidence in herself and strength in the marriage. Together she and her husband decided to try again for the child they so longed to have. Noelle felt confident that she had finally achieved the optimal physical, mental and marital state for conceiving a child. If it was not to happen this time, at least she felt she had done everything in her power to help her chances. This time, however, her prayers were answered. She conceived and carried to term healthy boy/girl twins. In looking back on her journey, Noelle believes that the work she did on herself taught her lifelong lessons on the importance of taking action in overcoming fears. You can have all the motivation, good intentions, and desire in the world but unless you take action, you will feel paralyzed by your fears and worry.

It Only Gets So Bad Before It Gets Better

You have probably heard the saying, "Is the glass half empty or half full?" a million times before. It relates to the idea that our attitudes play a big role in determining whether we feel mostly sad or mostly happy, mostly fulfilled, or mostly dissatisfied. Although conceiving a child is a process that is out of our control, there is one piece that we can own and that's our attitude. Let's take this a step further and see how the natural laws of the universe might affect our ability to deal with loss, disappointment, or a bad attitude regarding conception of a child.

Have you ever noticed that when you walk into a forest you can only go so far before you start walking out? It can only get so dark at night before it starts to get light again. When you ride in an elevator you can't go any lower than the bottom floor before the elevator starts to ascend again. The winter can only last so long until it becomes spring and the spring becomes summer and the summer becomes fall.

Life is constantly changing and moving. Remember in the OM chapter when we talked about the t'ai chi symbol? This is the very concept it represents: you can only go so far one way before you hit the end or start going in another direction. We find this extremely helpful when dealing with disappointment or loss because it hints at the idea that we will feel really, really bad for just so long before we start to feel good again. For some of us the feeling bad part could last a long time but, as time and the flow of the universe continue to move, we will eventually come out of the darkness and back toward the light.

This is one reason why the solstice is such a powerful time to set new intentions. In the Northern Hemisphere the winter solstice, which occurs around December 21 every year, is the time when the sun is at its greatest distance from the celestial equator. That means it's the shortest day of the year; the day with the most darkness. After the solstice, the light begins to return and the days start getting longer. What great symbolism for starting something new or letting go of something that doesn't serve us anymore. In fact, both the winter and summer solstices and their corresponding change of seasons can bring great energy and power behind your intentions. Generally speaking, the solstices occur around the following times: December 21 (winter) and June 21 (summer). The equinox occurs March 21 (spring) and September 22 (fall) and occurs when the sun crosses the plane of the earth's equator and day and night are of equal length. This is an auspicious time for finding balance or balancing out the imbalances in your life.

WEEK 7 ACITIVITY: CLEARING RITUAL

This ritual can be done at your home to help rid negative thoughts or events that are causing you to feel loss, sadness, or disappointment. You will need a candle, pen or pencil, paper, music, water, sandalwood incense, sage stick, a flower, and a sacred symbol, picture or statue of a holy deity or thing that represents to you the feelings of love and healing.

Start by finding a space in your home that will offer you complete privacy, peace, and good ventilation or a window for the sage portion of the ritual. Create a small, short altar that you can sit in front of. On your altar place a candle, the flower, the lit sandalwood incense, the sage stick, and a statue, picture or symbol of your holy deity. Dim the lights and lower your curtains so the flame of the candle glows visibly. Start your ritual by saying a prayer, meditating, or contemplating those areas of your life that need clearing. Ask your deity or symbol for assistance, love, and guidance through the process of clearing from your mind, body, and consciousness all the cobwebs of life that have you feeling stuck, sad, fearful, attached, or in a state of delusion. This is your ritual so take as long as you like surfacing your feelings and giving them to your deity or symbol of love and healing.

Next, with your pen and paper, begin to write a letter or message to anyone or anything with whom you would like to communicate. Allow your deity or sacred symbol to create a bridge between you and other planes of existence. If you lost a child through miscarriage and need to commune with that child, write him/her a letter. If you feel that you need guidance from a relative, saint, or sage who is no longer on this earth, write him or her a letter. If you feel your greatest healing will come by writing a letter to yourself, then write it. The purpose of this exercise is for you to be able to articulate and write down those feelings that are held deep within. Again, we are surfacing and clearing obstacles, afflictions, and feelings that are blocking the path to our true happiness.

When your letter is finished fold it and place it near you, play soft, relaxing, or meaningful music, and just sit with your thoughts. Next, begin to softly gaze into the cool part of the flame of the candle for a few minutes. Gazing of this nature is considered a form of meditation in and of itself. If this feels uncomfortable on your eyes, look just above or just below the flame. Now close your eyes and imagine that you are breathing the flame in through your nostrils and bathing every part of your body with it. In your mind's eye, envision it burning away negative thoughts, feelings, and emotions and removing darkness, from within you so only light remains. Imagine that as the light of the flame becomes wider and brighter, it sends off its healing power to those around you so that you can be a light for them, too.

When you feel the time is right, take the sage stick from your altar, light it, and then blow out the flame so that only the smoke stream is left. Use the smoke stream from the sage to outline your entire aura. Start with your feet and then move all the way up toward your head and back down again on the other side. In some Native American cultures it was believed that smoke like this helped lift negative thoughts so that they could be carried away toward the sky and offered to the Great Spirit. With this in mind, purify yourself symbolically with the sage and then douse the sage lightly in the water or smother it in a fireproof bowl. The clearing ritual is now complete. You may choose to save your letter or, better yet, burn it safely in your fireplace or backyard fire pit and let the words from your message be carried by the smoke up to the Great Spirit.

Letting Go of Your Negative Attitudes and Thoughts

IN A STUDY of women undergoing IVF procedures, researchers asked the question: "Does stress affect fertility and pregnancy rates?" The researchers looked at whether stress from a patient's life situation or stress from the procedure negatively reduced the patient's ability to achieve pregnancy or to have a live birth. The women were given questionnaires to rate their moods, feelings about infertility, expectation of achieving pregnancy, amount of social support, coping style, and overall stress levels. The questionnaires were completed at their first clinic visit, before and after hormone use and before embryo transfer. The results showed that women who had higher expectations of achieving pregnancy had less overall stress, had a greater number of eggs retrieved and fertilized, a higher number of embryos to transfer, and a higher pregnancy rate as compared to the women who had a lower expectation of pregnancy and a higher rate of stress. (*Klonoff-Cohen* et al, 2001)

How to change negative attitudes

This study is just one piece of information that supports the idea that how we look at our ability to conceive a child and our overall attitudes can play an important role in our fertility. This is not to say that negative thinking causes infertility. It may not affect our reproductive biology, but negative thinking can lead to stress, anxiety, or depression, which as already discussed have been shown to adversely affect pregnancy rates. We cannot help but think there is some wisdom to the idea that changing the way you think about your fertility can have a profound impact on your overall happiness and sense of well-being. Regardless of your conception challenges, you still have freedom of choice. You can choose whether you want to go through fertility being happy or whether you want to go through fertility being negative and sad. Remember that our perceptions are indeed our realities.

Tami writes:

I used to visit St. Louis, Missouri, quite frequently when I had my corporate job. I never really liked it. It always seemed kind of dark and dingy and I remember thinking that there weren't enough good hotels, restaurants, or shops in town for visitors to enjoy. About a year after I had decided to quit my job, my husband and I traveled to St. Louis to attend a wedding for a dear friend. While driving in our rental car past the city, I noticed that the sky was particularly blue that day and that St. Louis looked really vibrant. We passed some of the old areas I used to frequent and noticed that there were all kinds of restaurants and cute little shops that had popped up. I motioned to my husband to look at all the great new places but he said they had all been there for quite some time. Apparently I had never noticed them before.

We checked into our hotel room and decided to spend the afternoon roaming around town. We had a delicious meal and then spent some time walking around, enjoying the small boutiques and antique stores that lined the street. I couldn't believe how much St. Louis had changed in just one year. As soon as that thought entered into my mind, I realized I was making a terrible mistake. It was not St. Louis that had changed, it was I who had changed. By not looking at St. Louis as the dreaded place where I had to spend my work day, my entire attitude shifted. I now saw St. Louis through the eyes of a tourist who was on vacation and it looked completely different. You see the change was not out there like I thought it was. The change was in me. This was a profound moment for me because I realized that just by changing your attitude, you can change your perceptions of life.

EXAMINE YOUR ATTITUDES

What is your attitude about your fertility? Is it dark and dingy like St. Louis? Are you missing beautiful parts of yourself or simply not noticing them because you are too busy feeling miserable and deficient? During our Tools for Healing class at PDtM, we ask women to describe their fertility and the fertility of their partner or spouse. It is amazing to hear the negative words they use like broken, barren, or dysfunctional. Why is it that we choose to shift our attitude from feeling truly vibrant and beautiful to feeling really deficient and broken? Remember, the more we feed these negative thoughts, the more they will grow.

Your thoughts can be compared in many ways to plants in a garden. There are the positive thoughts that can be represented by the tulips, which are pretty but fragile, or the roses, which are fragrant but thorny. The weeds are like negative thoughts which just plain old get in the way. They are the worst of all the plants because, left unattended, they grow out of control. You have to pluck them by the root to get rid of them because, if you're not careful, they will start to choke out the fragile tulips and beautiful roses. Remember the kleshas from the last chapter? Those suckers are at the root of your negative thoughts. Ironically, the flowers also take a great deal of care. You have to water them, make sure they get enough sunlight, stake them upright and maybe even fertilize them. Every day, you need to tend the garden of your mind. Pluck out the negative thoughts, words, and feelings by the root. If you don't, they will grow like weeds and begin to take over even your most positive thoughts. Your mind does not like to be void of thoughts. Even when you try to quiet it, those thoughts will keep spinning around in your head. Be diligent in staying after those weeds.

At PDtM we have met women who are approaching their fifth and final round of IVF who have said, "If it doesn't happen this time, I know I will be okay. I will have the child I am meant to have." Similarly, we have had patients who fall apart after their first unsuccessful IUI because they have convinced themselves it will never happen. Now, you might argue that everyone has a different tolerance for pain and varying circumstances, which make their situations unique. However, time and time again, we have seen that the patients who have spent time learning about themselves, caring for their holistic well-being, and keeping a balanced attitude are almost always better equipped to handle the fertility journey.

If you are having difficulty getting pregnant, how has this affected your ego and sense of self? How has it affected your spouse's or your relationship together? Perhaps you are among the many who are finding that the stresses associated with infertility and IVF treatment are having a negative impact on your psychological health and marital quality? (*Wang* et al, 2007)

WEEK 8 ACTIVITY 1: BELIEVING YOUR LIES

There is an old belief in yoga philosophy that the root cause of all of our suffering comes from each of us believing in three lies. So what are your lies? What have you come to believe that is actually causing you to live in a world made up of false perceptions and ideas? Write them down. Then ask yourself the following questions:
• Are they true?
• What emotional reactions do you have to these lies?
• How are these emotions serving you or not serving you?
• What would your life be like if this thing were untrue or you didn't think this thought? Could it change your perception of the world or even yourself?

Svadyaya

When you begin your exploration of self, you actually begin the second step of the Kriya Yoga path we described in the introduction. This step is called "*svadyaya,*" a Sanskrit word that translates as "self-study." It is a process whereby we begin to look deep inside ourselves to more fully understand our attitudes, beliefs, and habitual patterns. It is not the process of obsessing: of grabbing hold of an idea and preoccupying the mind with it. It is more the process of unlearning all the negative things we have conditioned ourselves to believe.

Self-conscious awareness is the first step in the process of self-study. Usually it is awareness that there is a problem in the way that you are thinking, like the realization Tami had that it was her attitude that had changed, not St. Louis. You might have awareness that the garden of your mind is full of weeds. Have you ever found yourself saying or thinking any of the following: "I'm never going to get pregnant." "My husband must not love me anymore because I can't conceive." "Life will be different if I have a child." More than likely, these are erroneous, "weedy" thoughts that you need to pluck from your mind.

WEEK 8 ACTIVITY 2: STUDYING YOUR ATTITUDES

Here is an exercise that will help you begin to study some of the attitudes you may have about your fertility. Answer the questions in your own personal diary or journal. When you are finished, go back and ask yourself if some of your stressors are based on false perceptions or ideas you have about yourself, your partner or your physician.

- What words would I use to describe my fertility?
- What words would I use to describe my husband/partner's fertility?
- What physical symptoms does my body experience through this process?
- How do I feel about my body?
- Do I exhibit any addictive behaviors or bad habits? To what am I addicted?
- What time of day do I most feel stress?
- Does having a child scare me in any way or make me feel uncertain?
- What is my relationship with my physician? Can I speak to him/her freely?
- Do I trust my physician?
- Do I trust myself to make all the right decisions? Why or why not?
- How does trying to conceive affect my marriage or relationship with my partner? My family? My friends?
- What are my dreams? In other words, where do I hope I will be 10 or 20 years from now? Can I visualize this future both with and without children?

DEVELOP YOUR AWARENESS

After you have identified the problem with the way that you are thinking, you need to bring awareness into the idea by saying, "I am aware that I am thinking _____." Like "I am aware that I am thinking my husband must not love me anymore because we do not yet have a baby." Then, ask yourself why you think this is so, "Why do I think my husband doesn't love me any more?" Remember, we are looking for the "root" cause here so you have to be honest with yourself. Now, write down your answers and then meditate upon each. Finally, ask yourself how you might feel if you changed your attitude about the situation. For instance, what if you focused on all the ways your husband shows you he loves you rather than the ways you think he doesn't? Could this kill the weed? Could it change your relationship with your spouse or, at the very least, thin out your garden a little bit so the roses can bloom?

Finding the root cause of our suffering is never easy. We need to start studying ourselves and bringing awareness into our thought process so that we can learn who we really are. Most importantly, we need to study ourselves to learn that we control our destiny, we control our lives and we have the ability to decide if we are going to live in the world as a happy person or as a sad person, as a person with a fertile mindset or an infertile mindset.

UNDERSTAND YOUR THOUGHT FORMS: CITTA

"In the province of the mind, what one believes to be true either is true or becomes true"

JOHN LILLY

In the world of yoga, it is believed that what we think and believe creates our reality. Here is a story from Tami's teaching experience that illustrates this point.

Tami writes:

Several years back we were teaching Yoga for Fertility to a packed room of both men and women at a doctor's office. I had had a really bad day. Lots of things were going on with the business, the kids were being particularly demanding and heading out the door at 6:00 p.m. to teach a yoga class was met with evil stares by my husband who seemed to need a bit of TLC himself that day. When I arrived at the venue to teach the class, I noticed a couple in the back of the room who seemed new to yoga and a bit unprepared for the class. Once we began the Yoga for Fertility class, the husband began to repeat every instruction I gave as if to mock the very words coming from my mouth. When I said, 'Squat down to bring blood flow into the uterus,' he would turn to his wife and in a very loud voice say, 'bring blood flow into the uterus.' Not only was his mocking disruptive to the class, it was disruptive to me. Each time I gave an instruction for a posture, he proceeded to repeat it in a loud and surly manner which had me thinking that I truly must be the worst yoga teacher on the planet. I began to wonder why I said the things I said. Coming from my mouth and then hearing the words repeated by him made me realize how stupid I sounded. To make matters worse, after he repeated everything I said, his wife would stare at me with big eyes as if she were watching and criticizing my every move. I felt the eyes of the entire class upon me, waiting, judging, and anticipating my next move. My self-esteem was being called into question right there in that class and I began to think all kinds of thoughts. I wondered why I had ever decided to be a yoga teacher. I questioned why I had decided to quit my well-paying corporate job and I wondered if I really had the time and energy to devote to this Yoga for Fertility business. Could I really make a difference in someone's life? Surely, this couple did not seem to be benefiting from what I had to offer that night. During the 90 minutes that I taught yoga that night, I began to imagine life without my business, without teaching yoga, and without the added stress of wondering if all my students were truly getting what they needed from my class. For a moment I thought maybe it was time to throw away the dream.

When the class ended, the couple from the back of the room started walking toward me. I braced myself and prepared for the worst, only hoping that their scorn and ridicule of the class would not be heard by the rest of the students who were, by now, packing up their yoga mats and heading for the door. The gentleman approached and said, "We really enjoyed this class and want to sign up for more. We want to make sure, however, that it would be okay since my wife is hearing impaired and I need to repeat the instructions so she can hear. She reads lips pretty well, though, as long as she can follow you with her eyes."

I don't think that couple ever realized what a huge impact they had on my life that night. They had taught me a very big lesson. I had created my negative reality based on the thoughts that were floating around in my head. I had come to believe something that not only was untrue it was completely illusionary. What if I had left class that night and decided to alter the course of my life? What if I had quit teaching yoga or stopped running PDtM or decided I was not worthy in some way? Would I have been right in the way I was thinking? No! Would I have been reacting to the erroneous thoughts in my head? Yes!"

In yoga there is a name for these incessant thoughts that run through our brain every day. They are called *"citta"* or mind stuff and these thoughts create the illusion (*"maya"*) that is our life. It is an illusion because we start to believe that everything we think is true so, therefore, our thoughts shape our reality. By changing the way we think, we can change our reality. Just remember the example of the yoga class with the woman who was hard of hearing. Tami's reality was that she must not be a good teacher based on the reaction of a couple in the back of the room. The truth was, the couple was dealing with a hearing disability and were trying to get the most out of the class. So what's the truth? The truth is anything you believe.

Thought Forms

Our thoughts can be our best friends or our worst enemies. In yoga and some Eastern philosophies it is believed that thoughts actually radiate energy, color, frequency, and vibration. Every thought has a magnetic field. Your thought forms attract all the other thought forms that are similar in nature and they become magnetized to your aura. If you hold kindness in your mind, your aura will hold this kindness and attract other people's thought forms of kindness. The result: you will radiate and be surrounded by kindness. If you hold thought forms of sadness, defeat, and infertility in your mind, you will attract more sadness, defeat, and infertility. Have you ever been around a really depressed person and then, after having spent some time with them, you, yourself, start to feel down in the dumps? That's because your aura is being bombarded by the negative vibration of their thought forms. Any little bit of negativity you have gets magnetized by theirs so you end up feeling rotten too. This illustrates the importance of surrounding yourself with people who have a higher vibration than your own. If you surround yourself with happy, smart, wise people, they will draw out of you the happy, smart, and wise parts of your personality. Your vibration will rise up to meet theirs. Unfortunately, this also suggests that you begin to rid yourself of relationships of low vibration that are energetically draining.

HARNESS YOUR THOUGHTS

Again, working with the power of thought forms is more than just positive thinking. It is shifting your attitudes to focus on what you truly want. Along the way you also have to feel worthy enough to receive it. It is the power of believing, with every morsel of your being, that you are fertile and will have the baby you so truly desire. By thinking fertile thoughts, you will attract fertility. If you are like many women who so desperately want a child and are having difficulty conceiving, you may find yourself avoiding situations where you might encounter babies or pregnant women. This, say many yoga gurus, is counterproductive to the fertility process. If you want a baby, they say, surround yourself with babies and pregnant women who are throwing off the vibration of babies and pregnancy. Expose yourself to them and allow those vibrations to be magnetized to your aura so that you are surrounded by positive and fertile pregnancy energy.

Not yet convinced? Here's another example of how citta, maya, and the power of thought forms can affect your life. Jackie works in an office and feels rejected one day at lunch when she waves at the boss but the gesture is not returned. Jackie decides she is being ignored because she is taking a lot of time off for her fertility-related appointments. Since the boss is unmarried and has no children, Jackie is convinced the boss is insensitive to her situation. Jackie begins to fear that the boss may fire her for not being completely devoted to the job. Acting on these impulses, Jackie goes out of her way to avoid the boss in the office because she doesn't want any confrontations and she certainly doesn't want to have to explain her absences. The more Jackie avoids her employer, though, the more the boss seems to be seeking her out. Jackie is convinced she is being micro-managed because the boss is concerned over her commitment to the job and is looking for an excuse to fire her. Jackie becomes defensive when her employer speaks to her about her projects. The boss, on the other hand, begins to think that Jackie has a bad attitude and wonders why she is being avoided. The boss begins to wonder if Jackie is hiding something because she always looks so suspicious. She tries to assess if Jackie is overburdened by her workload but is met with defensive comments and evil stares every time she brings it up. The boss begins to resent Jackie's attitude and wonders why she is putting up with it given there are at least five other people in the office who would love to be promoted to her position. In the end, Jackie gets fired and her prophecy is fulfilled.

Here's another example. Have you ever known someone who was convinced their house was haunted because of the creepy vibe it emitted? Again, these are thought forms the owner is likely picking up from the previous owner/s. If someone died in the house, it is possible that the thought forms of sadness or illness still linger in the house.

BELIEVE IN YOUR FERTILITY

Perhaps you can think of several examples of how citta and maya play their hand in your desire to be a parent. We ask women in our Yoga for Fertility class to list on a white board all of the thoughts that enter their minds when going through the fertility process. As you might expect, many of them write the phrase, "This is never going to happen for me." If we begin to believe that it will never happen for us, chances are it will be very difficult. In yoga we say that in order for something to manifest into reality, you have to be able to imagine it first. If you can't imagine it, you can't create it. Again, that is because we draw into our lives that which we think about and believe in. Now you may say that you think about becoming a mother every single day, but the baby has yet to manifest. Here is the tough part; thinking about it is not enough. You have to truly believe that it will happen for you.

The trick is, however, you have to let the universe bring that child into your life in a way that is most harmonious for you. That is why you need to go "out of your mind." Often times, we focus on getting pregnant rather than on having the child. Our minds are busy imagining the day we get a positive pregnancy test, or when we get to tell our husbands the good news. We imagine watching our belly grow and then delivering a child that looks like our perfect clone. Our focus should shift to imagining the child we are meant to have. Think about being a parent and loving a child and let the universe take care of the rest. You will be amazed at the dramatic shift you will see in your personality when you stop trying to control the process of becoming a parent and focus more on the prize. You will attract that child like a magnet to a piece of metal.

EXERCISE COMPASSION

The biggest and most dreadful piece of citta you can have in your head is that you will never be a parent or that you are somehow unworthy. Quite a few students at PDtM have felt that their infertility is due to the termination of a pregnancy they had earlier in life. Somehow, they believe, God or the universe is dishing out "payback" for their actions. Deep down inside they feel unworthy and believe they are being punished for past transgressions.

If you find yourself in a similar situation, try practicing compassion. Compassion means that you understand that you made the best decision you could at that particular moment in time. Compassion means that you are able to share in your own suffering and see the woman who existed then and the woman who exists now are two separate people. As time goes on, we become wiser. How you make decisions at the age of 19 is very different from how you might make decisions at the age of 30. Why? You have gained 11 years of wisdom and experience, that's why. It is also very easy for us to forget the various circumstances that may have surrounded the events that caused you to make a particular decision. At any given point in time, an individual is making the best possible decision he or she can based on their life experience. That is compassion. Do not let these negative thoughts cloud your judgment or sense of self because, for most of us, they are completely false, they are avidya. Instead, find ways the world shows you compassion and from it learn to be kind to yourself.

Some yoga philosophers believe that before a child comes into her mother's life, the little soul first explores the mother's soul to see if they are compatible. The child makes sure that the mother has the karma necessary for it to accomplish its life's goals. It is thought that this is done by spinning up and down the mother's cerebral and spinal axis where the chakra system resides. If the karma is a match, the child chooses the mother. If the karma does not match, the child moves on to another soul. If the child has the karma of adoption, then it will wait to find the mother with the same adoption karma. If we look at childbirth from a very esoteric viewpoint, perhaps this process of karma matching is the very reason some pregnancies are never fulfilled or end in miscarriage. Either the karma of the two souls were not quite right or simply by inhabiting the mother's body for a short period of time, the karma becomes fulfilled for one or both beings.

Remember, if you want to be a parent, then one day you will be a parent, but you must be open to the way in which that will happen. When you are finally holding that child in your arms, it will be your child and you will be its mother, no matter how the two of you are brought to each other.

Tami writes:

When I was a sixth grader I remember my teacher saying that God always answers our prayers. He either says, "yes, no, or maybe." Growing up, I have tried to remember these words on more than one occasion when life was proving particularly challenging. For some reason it brought me great comfort to think that my innermost thoughts, desires, frustrations, or pains had somewhere to land. I have always felt that a benevolent God watches over me from a higher place and guides my every move with discerning answers of yes, no, or maybe.

Looking back, my struggles with infertility seem like an out-of-body experience. Who was I back then that I could not easily accept the answer "no" when my time for pregnancy had *not come, or "maybe" as I moved to the next round of treatment in the hopes of getting that baby? I can remember walking back from the doctor with my husband after one of my failed cycles of injectible meds. I was despondent that this more aggressive treatment had failed and said to Brian, "perhaps the answer is 'no.' Maybe we are just not meant to have a baby." I expected him to nod in agreement, reach out and hug me so we could both mourn the loss of our dream. Instead he said, "Tami, if we want to be parents, we will be parents. If we want a baby, then we will have a baby." What was he saying? My own husband was telling me the answer was "yes" when I had convinced myself God was telling me "no." Who was right? Was there even a right answer? I felt confused until I had this epiphany that what God and Brian were each telling me was exactly the same thing. I was just too dumb to hear it. "Yes" you can have a baby but "no" it might not be your biological child.*

That out-of-body experience came at the moment I realized I had to make a decision. I either wanted a baby or I didn't. I either had to play by the rules of the universe, or get left out of the game entirely. I could have what I wanted, but maybe not the way I imagined. What was my answer? What would I choose: baby or no baby? It was really as simple as that. You either want a baby or you don't, Tami. You either want to be a parent or you don't. Decide, but stop thinking that the answer has to come wrapped up in a bow in exactly the size and color you imagined in your head. All of this citta (mind-stuff) came into my consciousness during the walk back from the doctor with Brian. I knew the answer. I knew in my heart that I wanted the baby. "Yes," I told God. "Yes, I want the baby. Yes, I want to be a parent. Bring me that child in whatever way I am meant to receive it." That was it, I felt cleared. I had committed. No more waffling. No more wondering if I'd make a good mother, or if my job would suffer or if my marriage would be okay once children entered the house. No more indecision or wonderment, no more "maybes." The answer was "yes" and I knew it deep down in my heart. At that very moment I turned to Brian and said, "Yes, we will adopt if we cannot have children." He grabbed my hand and nodded in agreement. The very next cycle I conceived my twins.

WEEK 8 ACTIVITY 3: VISUALIZATION FOR THE CHILD YOU ARE MEANT TO HAVE

Lie down on your bed or on a soft surface. Take three long inhales and exhales and focus on the sound of your breath for four to five minutes until you feel relaxed. Now, imagine that your feet become as light as a feather and begin to hover above the rest of your body. Next, imagine both of your legs becoming weightless and beginning to float. Move toward your buttocks and navel. Imagine them lifting with great ease into the air to join your legs and feet. Now, imagine your entire torso is floating and then your arms. Finally, feel your head become as light as a feather so that your entire body is hovering above the ground in complete weightlessness. Imagine that you are now flying through a meadow of wild and fragrant flowers that opens into a giant, green, and fertile mountain range.

Imagine you are flying and dipping from canyon to peak of each mountain. At the top of one of the mountain peaks, see that there is a crowd of small children looking up at you. One of the children is waving at you and beckoning you to take him or her with you. Swoop down and pick up your child. Embrace him or her in your arms and then fly back into your body holding the child you are meant to have within you.

WEEK 8 ACTIVITY 1. COMBING YOUR AURA

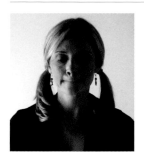

Feel like you've been bombarded with lots of negative thought forms lately? Try energetically cleansing your aura next time you are in the shower. Pull your top lip over your top teeth and pull it taut with your bottom lip until you feel like your nostrils are big and elongated. Exhale out with force and as you do so, pump the muscles in the abdomen. Quickly inhale through the nose and then continue to exhale forcefully again while pumping the abdomen until all the breath is spent. Quick inhales and forceful exhales will help comb your aura of its negative thought forms. Next, allow the water from the shower to take those thought forms down the drain. Cleanse your body with soap as usual. All clean now!

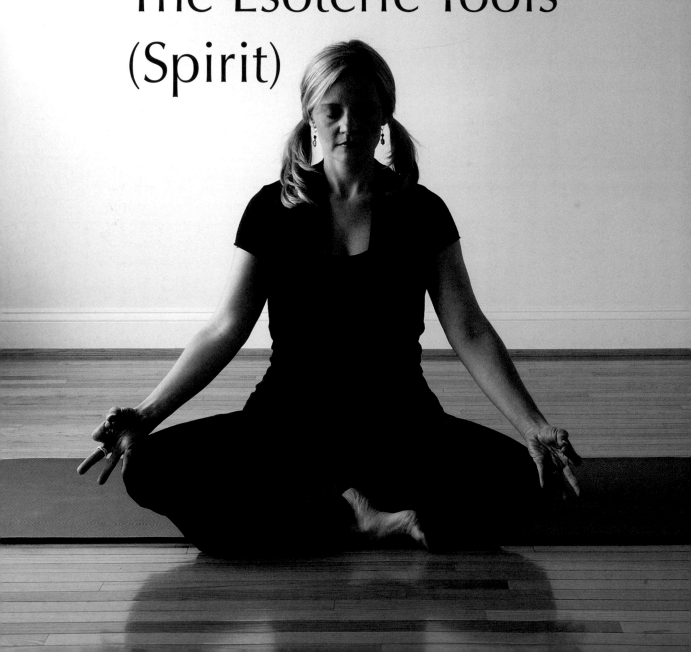

The Esoteric Tools (Spirit)

The Koshas: Giving Up Your Erroneous Definition of Self

"Let us not look back in anger or forward in fear, but around in awareness."

JAMES THURBER

Tami writes:

If you have ever visited a construction site, you may have noticed that before the actual foundation can be poured, the land must be surveyed and then excavated. The survey helps the builder get an overall picture of the project including the boundaries, elevations, and angles that must be observed. During the excavation process, the land is dug out in order to make a hole for the foundation. I watched one such project from my office window in Chicago several years back when a developer decided to turn a parking lot into a retail complex just across the street from where I worked. During the excavation process, they started turning up pieces of broken glass onto the soil. Apparently, the parking lot had been built atop an old light bulb factory.

Light bulbs contain phosphor coating dust, the toxic metal mercury and other chemicals, which the workers were afraid might be present on the newly excavated soil. It was feared that prolonged exposure to such substances could cause neurological damage and even cancer in humans. As a result, the entire development project was put on hold and an environmental abatement team was hired to clean the soil and get rid of any potential toxins. In came the equipment and human task force dressed in what looked like white space suits. They even had their own oxygen and air handlers attached to their headgear. It was a huge ordeal and great expense to the developer, not only in getting everything cleaned up but also an expense because of the huge amount of lost time on the project. A few months later, however, the foundation was poured and the building commenced. Today there's a nice grocery store, shops, and a movie theater where the old light bulb factory used to be. I often think about that developer and I'm convinced he sleeps better every night knowing that he did the right thing by cleaning up the toxins that could have potentially harmed other people. His foundation is now built on proper soil.

We share this story because it is a great metaphor for our own lives. At the surface, we all believe the soil of our mind is relatively clean. When we start to dig into the very fiber of our being, we begin to see some of the toxins hiding there. Some of these toxins are physical. These are the yucky things we feed our bodies; our ability or inability to maintain a healthy weight, get good sleep, or stop drinking and smoking. Beyond the actual meat and bones, we have attitudes about our bodies, our figures, and our face that determine whether ours is a body image of self-love, self-hate, or some sort of schizophrenic see-saw between the two. As we dig deeper, we notice toxins in our mind that have shaped our reality, our personality, and our attitudes. Finally, we begin to see the more existential side of ourselves. We begin to evaluate our self-worth, our relationship with God, and our interconnectedness to the universe. The deeper we excavate, the more "stuff" seems to come up. Pretty soon we realize that by uncovering these toxins we have to deal with them. We can either cover them back up with soil or excavate and abate them forever.

When we first started teaching yoga at PDtM, it became clear that yoga asana, the most obvious component of yoga for fertility, was simply scratching at the surface. In some cases yoga asana even stirred up physical toxins to the point that women were actually turned off: "I'm too fat for yoga," or "I'm too inflexible," or "I'm uncoordinated," were just some of the toxins that bubbled up. It became clear that if we were serious about promoting the use of yoga for fertility, we'd have to provide a healing framework that allowed for the excavation of toxins in a safe and healing way. In fact, it's this process of excavation and abatement that we believe is the most important step toward conceiving a child and finding happiness in life. As we mentioned in the introduction, the ancient yoga sages provided us with a philosophical method for looking at how to start this delicate process of "cleaning the soil of our lives." They claimed that each one of us has five different sheaths or envelopes surrounding our spirit, called "koshas."

What are Koshas?

If you have ever done yoga before, you probably know (or have heard) that it promotes well-being on many different levels. From the Western perspective it is common to say that yoga is a "mind-body" modality because it helps heal the physical body and calms the mind. Yoga therapy is even more specific on this point. In this view, human beings are believed to have five *different* bodies, called koshas, which provide a wonderful road map for self-study and healing. Different yogic techniques promote health and awareness in each of these bodies. Thus, the ultimate aim of *all* yoga practices is the healing and integration of the koshas, and the creation of "whole being health." This theory of the koshas was first presented in written form in the Vedantic scripture called the *Taittriya Upanishad* (about 1,000 BCE). This model is used extensively in yoga therapy traditions even today and we think it is a great key in helping you understand more about your mind, body, and fertility.

So, you may be asking how does the kosha model heal infertility or aid with conception? This is a question we put to our students at the beginning of each new class session at PDtM. To answer the question, it is important to first understand that each of us lives in two different worlds: an outer world and an inner world. Let's take a moment to explore exactly what these concepts mean in the context of our day-to-day existence.

OUTER WORLD
Put simply, our outer world consists of our body and our mind. This world feels pain, gets stressed out, wants to control its destiny, and is always changing. The fact that we cannot control it nor predict life's changing events creates even more stress and uneasiness in this world because the mind longs for the familiar, even if it is bad. Since this world is largely controlled by our thought process, it is always looking for something to think or worry about. It is absorbed in endless mind chatter (citta). It obsesses over the past and feels fearful about the future. This outer world is pretty straightforward. It comprises all the mental, emotional, and physical stress and discomfort we feel each and every day.

INNER WORLD
Our inner world, in contrast, is a bit more difficult to define. A yoga guru once told this story: As a young boy he had a dream that he was surrounded by deities from all the world's religions. There was Jesus, Krishna, Buddha, Abraham, Allah, saints and sages of all religions. Standing before them, the boy announced in his dream, "Will the real God please come forward?" With that question, each of the deities stepped forward and said, "I am God." Each then converged into one point of energy or light and then receded back into their Divine forms again.

YOUR DIVINITY
You see, no matter what name you give it—we prefer God, but you might see it as Universal Energy, Cosmic Consciousness, Spirit, Soul, or the Void—it is all the same. From this very bindu or ball of light is manifest all of creation. Each of us, and all living things contain the spark of "Divinity." We are not children of the Source or God, we are brothers and sisters, projections of the Source. Although we are externally imperfect, we contain the seed of perfection. You are in God and God is in you and when you do not recognize your own

divinity, you cannot recognize the divinity in the world. Conversely, when we do not acknowledge the Divinity in others, we cannot see it in ourselves. That is why, at the end of yoga, we say "Namaste." It literally means, "The Divine/Light in me bows to the Divine/Light in you." You've probably heard or read this saying before, "We are spiritual beings having a physical experience, not physical beings having a spiritual experience." When we accept this statement, we have come a step closer to connecting with our inner world which is the world of the most profound healing. The part of us that perceives this truth is called the "Witness" because it watches our mind and body act out the drama of our everyday life. At PDtM we believe that any healing that occurs, outside of the valuable effects of relaxation, good nutrition, exercise, and proper sleep, is the result of a greater awareness of the Witness world within us.

It is believed that when one connects with the Witness, they will find true bliss or happiness. They are able to transcend the outer world and its attachment to negative self-image. Unfortunately, the Witness eludes all but the most enlightened of souls and it may take more than just a few sessions of yoga and acupuncture to connect with it. Let's just say that connecting with Spirit can take a lifetime (or several if you believe in reincarnation). Perhaps, though, you have connected with this part of yourself at some time in your life, if only for a brief moment. Have you ever experienced a time when suddenly, for no reason, you felt extreme happiness and bliss? For those few seconds, everything seemed right with the world and you felt as if you had been handed the key to the universe? Your senses become heightened and you may even get a chill up your spine or goose bumps on your skin. Your heart feels an overwhelming sense of love and contentment. Suddenly, as quickly as it came, the feeling dissipates.

These momentary connections with the Witness remind us that it does exist. It is not a state of intelligence, thinking or mental aptitude, it is a feeling state. You feel, deep within yourself, that you are a part of the world, not apart from it. It's as though the zoom lens in your mind pulls back and is able to see that all is right with the world, and most profoundly, that all is right with *you*.

SPIRIT

Ancient sages tell us that "Spirit," in its perfect state, wants to have human experiences and so chooses to inhabit a physical body and acquire a mind and so becomes the Witness. The Witness is never lost, it simply gets covered by layers of mind and body issues that make it difficult for us to remember what true freedom is really like. The Spirit is hidden under the five koshas, similar to lampshades around a light bulb. The more you peel away the lampshades, the brighter the light becomes, until nothing but pure, radiant light remains.

Koshas and Healing

It is believed in many yoga therapy models that an illness can arise from separation at the level of one or more of the koshas. The first tool in healing is awareness. This awareness comes from the mental and physical connection you make that something is out of balance. As you work to integrate body, mind, and spirit, the healing process can be spontaneous and even effortless.

Disease

At PDtM, we do not view infertility as an "illness." Nor do we ascribe to the belief that a woman who has difficulty conceiving is "broken" and needs to be "healed." However, many women participate in unhealthy habits, stress, erroneous thinking, and physical imbalances, which can contribute to reproductive dysfunction. These habits could also contribute to heart disease, cancer, or diabetes. We believe it is important to look at all aspects of our constitution to assist with the healing process. Although trained in anatomy and physiology, a physician might differ greatly from a holistic practitioner in how they approach healing in the body. A physician may know everything there is to know about bones, organs, ligaments, and tissue; however, they may not be truly interested in your physical, emotional, mental and spiritual self. The holistic practitioner or yoga therapist may probe for information that Western medical systems regard as extraneous including your emotional state, spiritual life, and belief systems. Let's look at a case study of how infertility can be treated holistically through the koshas.

The Origin of Disease

The origin of disease begins at very subtle levels and filters down into the more gross or physical levels. For example:

- Bliss body: *When you feel separated from faith, or the source of spiritual connection that gives you peace and clarity regardless of what else is happening, illness can manifest in this most subtle body.*
- Wisdom body: *Illness in this body is like seeing the world through colored glasses (good or bad) instead of clear ones. When your view is obscured you are unable to recognize your own innate wisdom.*

- Psycho-emotional body: *Mental pain and anguish cause disease in the psycho-emotional body. This occurs when we are unable to see that we are not our thoughts.*
- Energy body: *The mental pain and anguish described above create blockage of prana or chi in our energetic body.*
- Physical body: *With an imbalance of chi or prana, physiological symptoms may manifest in the physical body, resulting in bodily pain, discomfort, and/or disease states.*

Ardel's Story: Kosha healing (Part 1)

Ardel was a 32-year-old woman who had been married for several years before trying to have children. She had imagined herself being a homemaker and mother to four or five kids so, with this goal in mind, she quit her job shortly after getting married. After trying to conceive for nearly a year, her first pregnancy ended up ectopic. This resulted in the loss of one of her fallopian tubes. When her case was further reviewed by a doctor, it was determined that the second fallopian tube would also need to be removed, due to scar tissue. This meant that Ardel would never be able to conceive a child without the help of a doctor and Assisted Reproductive Technology (ART).

Ardel had heard stories about other women losing tubes to STDs. She had never been promiscuous, but in her state of self-blame and doubt she wondered why this could possibly have happened to her. She wanted to turn to a higher power, but Ardel grew up in a household that, for the most part, was not religious. There was not the support of faith, church or a spiritual teacher to whom she could turn with this irrational sense of guilt. This made her unsure about how to pray or connect with God in a way that would be healing. The very foundation of Ardel's belief system began to crumble, thus affecting her bliss body consciousness. Although she had always imagined God to be merciful and forgiving, she could not help but feel as though she was estranged and disconnected from Spirit.

Was her dream of children to be shattered? If she was not to be a mother, then what was she to be? She had planned her entire life around the idea of having and raising children. Ardel began to doubt her worthiness and ability to be a mother. She was now unable to see clearly. Ardel began to project her feelings of guilt and inadequacy upon her marriage. Although she was well supported by her husband, she felt as though she had failed him. When her first attempt at in-vitro fertilization was not successful, she found herself getting moody and depressed. Ardel's Psycho-emotional Body was now experiencing a great deal of mental pain.

In time, Ardel's medical treatments were requiring more time, cost, and emotional resiliency. With each "failed" cycle, she found herself spiraling downward. Ardel was not able to sleep, she began eating poorly and became lethargic and disinterested in those activities which formerly brought her great joy. Ardel began to lose more prana, the life-force energy that fuels our physical, mental, and spiritual being. Her chakras and energy channels were becoming increasingly blocked as her dream of having a child eluded her.

Not surprisingly, Ardel found herself in the hospital with terrible head pain. The doctors struggled to find out what was causing the excruciating discomfort and found irregularity in her blood work. Since further testing and potential surgery were indicated, Ardel's subsequent IVF cycle was cancelled, confirming her belief that she was broken in every way.

Healing

This story clearly illustrates how an imbalance in the anandamaya kosha (Bliss Body) can ultimately affect all the koshas, resulting in physical disease. In order to rebalance the koshas, it is necessary to work in the opposite direction; from the bottom up so to speak. To "fix" our energy body we must first work through the physical. To reach the level of our thinking, we must first learn to control our breath. That is why breathing is such an important aspect of fertility treatment. If you have any stress, anxiety, or feel highly emotional about the fertility process it is unlikely that these symptoms will be controlled unless you first learn to nurture your body (annamaya) and your breath (pranamaya). This can be a simple process like raising your arms overhead and stretching for five minutes and then sitting down quietly and taking long, slow, even breaths. Deep, rhythmic breathing is extremely useful for fertility and can, quite literally, change the momentum of the mind. We will talk more about this in an upcoming chapter. Penetration of these first two koshas can also come through deeper work like psychotherapy or meditation. The point is, that even if we are consciously unaware that the work is happening, all healing is self-healing and it is healing that must exist chronologically through the koshas.

So, if we are ultimately our own healers, is this to say that medicines like antibiotics, for instance, are not real cures for diseases like a bladder or sinus infection? No. There is scientific evidence that supports the fact that antibiotics can attack and kill certain bacteria in the body. But what caused the bladder infection? Are we run down, over-stressed, eating poorly, and sleeping little? Have all of these things made us more susceptible to these afflictions? Think about what happens when we get the flu. Our bodies literally shut down and go to sleep for a day or two. We throw up and have diarrhea in an act of detoxification. Have you ever tried being really worried about something going on at work when you have a fever of 102 and can't lift your head from the pillow? The fever somehow melts away our external stresses, doesn't it?

Can each one of us control whether or not we have the ability to conceive a child? PDtM says probably not, scientists would say definitely not. Both of us would agree, though, that we can control *how* we react to our struggles with infertility. We may not be able to determine if we will get pregnant or when, but we can determine what steps to take in order to heal the physical, mental, and spiritual symptoms of infertility and the first step is kosha awareness.

Ardel's Story: Kosha healing (Part 2)

So let's return to Ardel. Her first step toward healing was the realization that she alone had the ability to heal all aspects of her disease. To get better, she knew she had to act on this realization and thus set off on a path toward self-discovery and healing.

Ardel started by attending a class at PDtM called Tools for Healing. This particular class focuses a lot on the mental and spiritual aspects of infertility and provides yoga tools for digging deeper into their root causes. Through visualization and meditation, Ardel realized two things: first, she needed to address the problem of her broken body and, secondly, she needed to be shown how to reconnect with God. Ardel committed to a regular yoga asana practice and began acupuncture for fertility treatments to help heal the physical body. Simultaneously, she received spiritual guidance with the intent of learning how to pray. As soon as she began a daily practice of prayer, something magical happened. Her head pain subsided and her blood work all came back normal. Rather than rush ahead with her next IVF cycle, Ardel chose to wait to ensure that healing on all levels of her being was optimal. About two months later, once she had reconnected with her Witness consciousness and felt empowered (rather than broken by her struggles with infertility), she called her doctor and scheduled an IVF cycle. Ardel subsequently conceived, had a healthy pregnancy, and gave birth to a baby boy.

It is next to impossible to decide one day that you need to move toward greater healing and, therefore, decide to "get in touch" with your Spirit. You cannot automatically connect like pushing a speed dial number on your cell phone. It takes a lot of effort and practice. In fact, the sages tell us that only by penetrating through each and every layer of the koshas are we able to progress in our meditation and truly understand the true nature of Self. We need to bring all the koshas into harmony, because when they are in harmony we have homeostasis and can begin to heal simultaneously on all levels. Remember then that the koshas do not exist independently from one another—they are interdependent. For example, your emotional state affects your health and the food you eat affects your vitality. By exploring these five sheaths, we become more in touch with our Spirit. We begin to yoke the physical, mental, and spiritual being into one balanced entity. This is the true definition of yoga, which comes from the Sanskrit word *yuj*, which means "to yoke." Yoga practices yoke—the process of uniting the Self with God.

WEEK 9: ACTIVITY 1: KOSHA EXPLORATION

Step 1

Get in touch with your physical body. Take your hand and grab a chunk of body, an arm, a thigh, a foot, maybe even a love handle. You may feel a bit strange doing this but this is your annamaya kosha. It is your skin, muscle, joints, bones, and organs, often referred to as the gross or dense body. Now, do a series of several yoga poses, like reaching up to the sky with your arms and swan diving down toward your feet. Hang in a forward fold, clasping onto opposite elbows. Do this several times and while you are doing it, focus all of your attention on what you are feeling and doing in your physical body. Feel the muscles work and the sturdiness of your bone structure. If you are tight, begin to feel a release in the body as you continue the series. When you are folding forward, feel the protrusion of the spine against the skin of your back. Touch your knee caps. Massage your shoulders.

Step 2

Next, incorporate breathing into your short series of yoga postures. As you sweep your arms up toward the sky, inhale deeply through the nose. Pause the breath for a second or two when your arms are fully extended over your head. When you swan dive forward, exhale through your nose. Spend some time inhaling and exhaling while you are folded in half. Focus on the sound of your breath then repeat the sequence. Notice how the flow of the breath joins the body to create a sort of movement dance. Breath and body flow in rhythmic unison. Congratulations, you have just explored your pranamaya kosha.

Step 3

Add this step to your series of yoga postures. Become aware of what you are thinking. Is your mind wandering off thinking about your "to do" list or what happened at work today? Turn back to your breath and turn all of your awareness to your inhales and exhales. If you begin to feel as though your mind is wandering, say to yourself, "neti, neti, neti" (pronounced netty, netty, netty). This means, "I am not this thought, I am not that thought, I am not thought." Repeat this mantra every time your mind begins to wander. As you begin to control your thought process, you will notice a new-found silence in your practice.

Step 4

After practicing steps 1–3 for at least five minutes, find a seat on the floor or in a chair. Close your eyes and keep your spine nice and straight. Turn your awareness back to your inhales and exhales, maintaining the mantra when needed. After a few minutes, drop the mantra and simply breathe. Notice that in between the inhale and exhale sound of your breath there is a moment of complete silence. In yoga it is believed that meditation is this point of silence or stillness of breath. Begin to enjoy these few seconds of breathlessness.

Step 5.

Maintaining your meditative position, begin to let go of all mantras and breathing techniques. Try to think of nothing, just enjoy the silence. When you feel like you are connecting with the peaceful and quiet side of yourself, ask yourself a question, any question. Now, listen to the answer. This answer is coming to you from your highest Self.

Learning the Value of the Breath: Pranayama

DO YOU FEEL like the fertility process has you constantly holding your breath? Each time you go to the bathroom at "that time of the month," do you hold your breath to see if you'll see the start of your period? How about when the doctor's office calls with an important result? We've seen patients who don't even exhale until they end their first trimester. Why is it that we hold our breath? In what way do we believe it will protect us?

Beth writes:

Breath-holding under duress is one of those things that we hold up as "just the way it is," and have long forgotten why we hold it to be true. Interestingly, I was handed the answer in a one-on-one encounter with a deer. My family was up in northern Wisconsin taking a drive through Peninsula State Park. We were driving slowly, enjoying the smells and the dappled sunlight on carpets of forget-me-nots. As the car turned around a bend in the road we came face-to-face with a juvenile white-tailed deer standing by the roadside eating the new spring leaves from a sapling. I stopped the car so we could look at the deer. She was standing completely still, every muscle tensed to run like the wind away from my car. And that's when I noticed that she was barely breathing!

We sat for about a minute, the deer looking at us and us looking back. As silly as it sounds, I tried to make eye contact and send her the telepathic "all's clear." A few moments later, her body relaxed and she continued on her path. Perhaps breath-holding is an ancient human defense against the unknown. Mystically, yoga teaches that breath retention equals the timeless state. Maybe our breath holding is an attempt to freeze the perception of safety in the current moment. With the next breath we must enter into the flow of time once again.

Yogic Breathing

Looking back to Chapter 2, we first discussed the importance of increasing the amount of life energy (qi or prana) in our physical system. In this chapter we'll go a bit deeper into the yogic perspective on breathing. This is really the first place in the book that we'll step into the more esoteric teachings of yoga. As you read on, you may feel yourself challenged to think outside of your comfort zone. We know many of the concepts presented here are esoteric, but we'll do our best to keep them relevant to the process of having a baby. It is our hope that as you keep your mind open to this ancient wisdom, you will find yourself moving into a place of healing that is beyond the physical.

It is a belief among many yogis that we are born into this world not with a certain number of years to live but with a certain number of breaths to breathe. After our last allotted breath is gone, the physical body dies. We suppose this theory is difficult if not impossible to prove through medical science; however, there is a study out of India that showed people who practiced slow breathing exercises for three months lowered sympathetic nervous system response and improved autonomic functions. (*Pal*, 2004)

Breath Control and Stress

You may recall from your biology class that the sympathetic nervous system is also known as the *fight or flight* mechanism. It is the body function that generally responds to physical and emotional stress by doing things such as increasing cortisol, heart rate, and blood pressure. It can also cause a change in digestive and respiratory functions, salivation, perspiration, and even the diameter of our pupils. When we experience prolonged periods of stress, this bodily system works overtime and we become a higher risk for heart disease, high blood pressure, weight fluctuations, and even depression. Given these dramatic effects on the body, then, it is not difficult to make the leap of faith that the faster we breathe, the sooner we may die from stress induced diseases. Learning to elongate your breath just may help you elongate your life—or have a baby.

Pranayama

Let's review a few terms before going further. In the kosha section of this book we learned that the second sheath or layer around our energetic anatomy is called the pranamaya kosha. The root word prana is a very important term in yoga. It is a Sanskrit word which refers to the amount of "life-force energy or vitality" that we have within us. Yama is control or restraint of this life-force. The word pranayama then, is the control or extension of life-force and is one of the eight limbs of yoga philosophy. It is believed to be heavily linked to Spirit. If someone feels confused or restless, it is likely that they have more prana outside of their body than inside. Too little prana in the body makes us feel stuck, restricted, or depressed. If we have not excavated out all the toxins or garbage that is within our body, prana is not able to completely fill it since there are already too many other obstacles occupying the space. Focusing intention and attention on getting negative stuff out and positive prana in is a vital part of overall health and fertility.

The concept of prana has been around for thousands of years and is mentioned in the sacred texts of India. The Japanese call it "Ki" and the Chinese refer to it as "Chi." We think Yoda and Darth Vader called it "the Force." Although we can acquire prana through breath work, prana is not oxygen or air because at the moment of our physical death prana leaves the body. If you were to pump oxygen into a dead body, it will not come back to life. The breath carries oxygen but it also acts as a mass transit system for carrying pranic energy into the body. Remember, our goal for fertility is to substantially increase the amount of prana we take in.

Efficient Breathing

If you are familiar at all with how modern-day homes are heated and cooled, you may know that in order for the air to reach every room of the house it must travel from the furnace or air conditioner through a series of ducts and then be funneled into each room via registers or radiators. Imagine that the air moving through this duct work is like a force that runs through your body, mind, and spirit. As it passes into each room, it cools or heats the room to just the right temperature. If the register is blocked by a heavy piece of furniture or if the duct work is clogged with dust bunnies, the air may not reach every room efficiently. Insufficient air means insufficient ability to regulate or balance the temperature of your house. As a result rooms become too stuffy, too hot, or too cold.

Similarly, our breathing process is a great metaphor for what we are feeling inside. Have you ever been in a traffic jam when you were late for work? Your respiration begins to intensify because stress causes the breath to become rapid and shallow. What about when you are scared? What happens to your breathing? Many of us hold our breath in anticipation of a frightening event. When we are relaxed and at ease our breathing might be slower and more mindful. When we begin to watch closely, we see that as life changes, our breathing changes, offering us a powerful opportunity for self-study.

Breathing for Fertility

For the purposes of becoming fully fertile, the breath is important for two reasons. On a physical level, breathing exercises can help lower cortisol levels, decrease heart rate, enhance relaxation, increase blood flow, and reduce pain. On a mental and emotional level, the mind influences how we breathe and, conversely, the breath influences how we think.

As we mentioned before, when we are upset, our breathing rate naturally increases but when we are relaxed, the rate of respiration decreases.

In the kosha model we discussed earlier, the pranamaya kosha or breath layer acts as a bridge between the body and the mind. If you really want to change the way you are thinking about your fertility or getting pregnant, you must first work through your body. You will need to exercise it, feed it properly, give it rest, and acknowledge that it is the only vehicle you have in which to transport your Spirit. You must locate any knots, resistance, or dust bunnies in the body and gently coax it back to balance. This is one of the great values of yoga postures or asana. It is a system or series of postures that allows us to explore our bodies in a gentle and mindful way, without force and without judgment. It allows us to remove the heavy furniture away from the registers and helps us clean out our duct work, so to speak.

Once this connection with body is achieved, it is important to learn breath control. For the advanced practitioner, breathing is a way to regulate different body functions. There is a breathing technique for inducing relaxation and one for creating stimulation. You can breathe kapalabhati (breath of fire) if you are too cold or sitali if you are too hot. Alternate nostril breathing can help bring about balance while bhramari (humming breath) can help clear head congestion. Again, the real purpose of breathing is to bring prana into the body. When there is a positive flow of prana, we are better able to relax and gain access to our minds.

Each of us has, in our life, had an encounter with prana. It is not visible but it can be felt and perceived. When the buds on the trees and shrubs are just bursting open in the new spring, that is prana. When you are about to sink your teeth into a red apple whose color, fragrance, and vibrancy seem to exude from the fresh, crisp fruit, that is prana. The smell in the air after a summer rainfall and the feeling it produces in you and in nature is prana. If you have ever felt really happy, healthy, or content but can't pinpoint why, it is likely an infusion of prana.

Techniques to improve your breathing

Choose one pranayama breathing technique from the selection below and begin practicing it everyday for at least five minutes. It is helpful to find a place in your home that is quiet, uncluttered, and does not have distractions like television, phones, or computers. The less "stuff" in the room, the less cluttered your mind will feel. Many people make the mistake of turning to breathing practices only when they are already in crisis or completely stressed out. This seldom works. You must learn to make a habit of breathing every day, even when you are not feeling particularly vulnerable or stressed. If we don't practice when we are happy and stress-free, we will not be able to sustain the practice when we really need it. It's like comparing breathing to your cardio-vascular well-being. You shouldn't just exercise and cut down on saturated fats after you have a heart attack; you should be mindful of what you eat and how you exercise long before you make a trip to the hospital. Then, perhaps, the heart attack won't happen.

For the purposes of trying to conceive a child, think of deep breathing practices as one of the most natural and holistic remedies you can use to relax or enliven your body. Try to let it be your first line of defense against stress or sluggishness in lieu of caffeine, sugar, nicotine, alcohol, sleeping pills, or other substances that are not appropriate during this special time in your life. You just may find that an addiction of the controlled breathing sort is a good addiction to have.

WEEK 10 ACTIVITY 1: BREATH AWARENESS

The purpose of this breathing technique is to help you attain better self-awareness of your physical and mental bodies. Simply find a comfortable seat on the floor or in a chair. Close your eyes and turn your attention to your breathing. As you inhale, say to yourself, "I am aware that I am breathing in." When you exhale say, "I am aware that I am breathing out." Repeat these phrases in unison with every inhalation and exhalation for at least five minutes.

If you are experiencing any physical pain, let's say cramping from your period or ovarian stimulation, find your breath through this breath awareness technique and then mentally send it to the afflicted area of the body. Imagine the breath numbing your pain like Novocain numbs a toothache. Every inhale brings in more Novocain or prana and every exhale sends it to the site of the pain for healing.

As you become more proficient with the technique you can use it in preparation for meditation. During the first stage of the breathing practice you will find heightened awareness of your mind and body and then you may experience a certain lifting sensation beyond the mind and body into deeper states of relaxation or meditation.

WEEK 10 ACTIVITY 2: EQUALING OUT
YOUR INHALES AND EXHALES (SAMA VRITTI)

When we are stressed-out we tend to breathe at a shorter, more rapid pace. When we are calm we breathe more slowly and deeply. This is a great breathing exercise to help change the momentum of your day and slow down your rate of respiration. The most difficult part is sitting down to do it when you may feel upset or like the world around you is very hostile. Remember, yoga and breathing are practices and that means they require a great deal of self-discipline.

While in a comfortable seated position with a straight spine and closed eyes, begin breathing through your nose. While breathing, mentally count to yourself like this: "Inhale

Ways to Increase Prana

Pranayama is not the only way to absorb life force energy although it is one of the easiest and most effective. Consider these other methods for absorbing prana into your subtle body, which then moves into your physical body:

- *Through the air you breathe: Take long walks and breathe deeply.*
- *Through the fluids you drink and foods you eat: Drink a lot of spring water and eat foods that are "alive." This means food should be fresh, organic, and not processed.*
- *Through good sleep: We don't have to do much of a sell job on this one. Just think about how you feel after a good night's rest versus how you feel when you pull an "all-nighter."*
- *Through natural sunlight: Allow your body to absorb the warm energy of the sun. Just make sure you remember your sun screen.*
- *Through your thoughts: Be pure of thought and action.*
- *Through laughter and joy: Did you ever notice how many times you take deep inhales and exhales during a good belly laugh? It's a breathing practice unto itself! Interestingly, researchers found that conception rates in women who were entertained by a clown before an IVF transfer had higher pregnancy rates. We are not the least surprised. After all, laughter = prana.*
- *Through yoga and ancient healing techniques like pranayama, hatha yoga, prayer, meditation, visualization, acupuncture, reiki, or massage. Pick one or even a couple that resonates for you and practice them daily.*

2, 3, 4, exhale 2, 3, 4; inhale 2, 3, 4, exhale 2, 3, 4." Keep breathing to this count for at least five minutes. Remember, if you start to feel dizzy or light-headed, stop the practice and return to normal breathing. At no time should the breath feel stressed or labored. Experiment a bit with the count. If inhaling and exhaling to the count of four proves too difficult, reduce the count to three. Similarly, if you feel the exercise should be lengthened, you can count to the number five with each round of breathing.

WEEK 10 ACTIVITY 3: THE HUMMING BREATH, BHRAMARI

In this breathing practice, you make the sound like a humming bee. It is useful for relieving stress, anxiety, depression, and anger. It is also believed to give you better mental clarity. Physically, it can help relieve headaches and congestion.

Inhale deeply through the nose. Exhale with a closed mouth and make a humming sound for the duration of your out breath. Inhale again through the nose and exhale while humming. Continue this pattern for at least five minutes. You can practice this breathing technique while in a restorative yoga posture such as Supta Baddha Konasana (see p. 150).

Seeing the Forest from the Trees: Meditation and Visualization

MOST WOMEN WHO are trying to have a child focus on just one thing: getting pregnant. What they don't recognize is that this type of obsessive focus can lead to imbalances in many different parts of their lives. In trying so desperately to nourish their physical fertility, attention to friendships, families, partners, careers, and self become choked by the process. As we learned in the kosha chapter, yoga invites us to broaden our focus enough to see that all things must "yoke" together in balance in order to create true happiness in life.

One-pointedness

This week we are going to use meditation to explore the concept of ascending the ladder of consciousness (one-pointedness). You may think you know all about this, being a conception guru, but as we just mentioned, the process of trying to conceive obliterates our sense of perspective. In this sense, it is one-pointed. Now, in this chapter, we are going to explore the idea of one-pointedness in a new way, the yoga way.

Francis' Story: Fertility Obsession

Francis Jones is a fertility patient. Every morning before her head lifts from the pillow she takes her basal body temperature. She's angry because it probably won't be accurate since she had to go to the bathroom an hour before she woke up. She eats the breakfast her nutritionist told her to eat, takes her prenatal vitamins, gives her husband a brisk kiss, and rushes out the door. Unfortunately, she forgets her palm pilot and briefcase since she is otherwise preoccupied. On the way to work she practices her affirmations. Her cell phone rings. Francis notices from caller ID that it's her sister, who has recently become pregnant and decides she can't handle that discussion just now and promises in her heart to call her back later. Guilt hits, but she promises she will call back.

When she arrives at work, she quickly rushes past her co-workers for fear they will ask why she left early yesterday. At least she remembered to wear her long-sleeved shirt which covers the bruises from her blood draws. Sitting at her desk she ignores the message light from her phone and turns to the computer where she begins her daily search for fertility blogs and checks the IVF boards. There's a pile of unopened mail and the in-box is overflowing, but Francis is just not motivated in her job anymore. Besides, she plans to quit when she has a baby, so why bother?

Francis is invited to lunch and manicures with some folks from the third floor but must decline because her acupuncturist could only see her at noon today. Her nails are a mess, her black roots are showing and she hasn't had time to get a pedicure in weeks.

There is a pit in her stomach about her husband's travel schedule. Didn't he say last night that he may need to go to Dallas on the 23rd? Didn't she tell him to keep that day free? He just doesn't get it. Man, what they could really use is a weekend away, together. Too bad the sex isn't even that great anymore.

Francis tells herself that she could really use a hard workout right now. Either that or a shot and a beer but we know that's not a possibility. Francis is having a really bad day. She wonders why life is always so difficult for her and knows that if only she could get pregnant everything would be as easy as pie.

Francis is a perfect example of fertility obsession or "one-pointedness." She only has eyes for one thing: getting pregnant. This should not come as a surprise to anyone, after all, that is how she managed to become Vice President in her office. She always believed you should never take your eyes off the prize. Now, in her mind, the prize is the baby and she will stop at nothing to achieve her goal.

Obsessing or one-pointedness in this sense can be very detrimental to Francis's overall health and well-being. While being committed to the process of getting pregnant can almost always pay off, it is necessary to find balance within the other aspects of life. In the scenario above, Francis encountered several acts of self-sabotage which will, ultimately, lead to increased stress, sadness, guilt, and separation. Let's see if we can find them. First, Francis woke up angry with herself for potentially ruining the accuracy of her basal body reading. Because her mind was split in a million different directions, she left the house without important tools for her work day. While in the car, she ignores the call from her sister that will, inevitably, haunt her with guilt later in the day. Francis shrugs her co-workers away at the risk of being excluded from office activities. Since these co-workers include both subordinates and managers, there is a certain anxiety that goes along with it. Will she be overlooked when the next promotion comes around? Francis is also feeling stressed because she rarely takes time for personal grooming and things she enjoys. Acupuncture feels great but she's not doing it for her health...she's doing it to get a baby. Now, with regard to her husband; Francis feels like this is a can of worms she can't even open. She finds her resentment keeps building month after month because he clearly does not understand what she is going through. More than anything, Francis just feels deprived. She feels deprived of caffeine, deprived of liquor, deprived of social interaction, marital attention, and good old-fashioned self-esteem. This is a great description of one-pointedness from a fertility perspective. It is that point at which you begin to wonder what is healthy determination and what is just a plain old obsession. As we all know, obsessions of any kind are never good.

A Yogi's Definition of One-pointedness

The yogis define one-pointedness much differently from Francis. In their viewpoint, one-pointedness is the desired outcome of years of meditation practice and self-discipline. It is one's ability to see that all things and all life contribute to one single thing — your overall happiness. In fact, there is an entire limb (of the eight limbs of yoga) which is dedicated to the practice of concentration and one-pointedness called "Dharana."

Now here's a metaphor to help explain the difference between Francis's one-pointedness and a yogi's. Francis's desire to get pregnant can be represented by many streams of water flowing out in various directions and ending in muddy pools filled with emotional pond scum. While she believes she is focusing on having a child, her energies are scattered in many, often negative, directions. A yogi has many streams of thought as well, but rather than flowing out into muddy pools, the energy converges and flows as a river into the clear ocean of her sacred intention.

Dharana is a necessary tool for meditation and happiness because it allows our minds to be focused on a single thought rather than a million thoughts. Unfortunately, Francis has chosen the wrong object of meditation. By focusing on having a child day in and day out, she is creating pain and suffering in her career, her relationships, her marriage, and her sense of self. Let us suppose for a moment that Francis changes her focus of meditation. Instead of pregnancy, what if Francis decided that her biggest goal in life was to be happy? What if all of her conflicts that she experiences every single day because of her fertility issues were now filtered through the lens of happiness? What if Francis was asked to think about and focus on those things that truly give her great joy? What would life be like?

Manifest Joy

The yoga philosophy tells us that our emotions and our thought process play a huge part in manifesting those things we want in our life. If we are focused on something that brings us joy, it is believed that joy will come to us. On the flip side, the more we feel "stuck" in our current existence, the more confined and miserable we will feel until the cycle is broken. This cycle can only be broken by you. Do not wait for your husband, your sister, your doctor, or a positive pregnancy test to change your life. Begin to positively change your life by focusing on all things that will bring you happiness right now. This might be a baby, but it might also be a BMW or a new nose. We honestly hope it's something less material, but it's okay if it isn't.

At PDtM we do an exercise called Seeing the Forest. One pitfall in the desire to have a child is that we become so consumed on having this baby, that we honestly begin to believe that all other aspects of our life will be made whole and happy upon its arrival. So we are going to expand our horizons beyond our noble desire of having a child, and think about what else might bring us happiness in five important areas of life: career; home; spouse/partner; personal growth and leisure; and family and friends.

Universal Laws

There are some universal laws that are important in helping us get what we truly want in life. One of the most important laws is that all things have energy, even our thoughts. Like energy, our thoughts do not simply leave our heads and die, they venture out into the universe like the sound waves from your radio. As our thoughts dissipate, they carry with them a frequency and vibration. This vibration becomes a magnet of attraction. It attracts back to us those things that we similarly think about or act upon. This concept ties into another universal law that many of you are familiar with: the Law of Karma or Newton's Law. This law states that for every reaction there is an equal and opposite reaction, or better said, what you sow is what you reap. When you send out vibrations of love, love will return to you. When you send out the vibration of fear, fear will manifest back in your life. That is why our minds and the way we think are so instrumental in helping us get what we really want out of life. Once we learn how to harness the spirit of these laws, we begin to tap into the field of creation that is present in each and every one of us.

Practicing Universal Law

There are seven major ways we can begin to practice these laws and bring positive change in our lives. They are as follows:

1. Change your attitude.
2. Be aware of ego attachments and the label you give yourself.
3. Be prayerful and express gratitude every single day.
4. Practice giving and selfless service. Expect nothing in return.
5. Go out of your mind. You create your own reality and often your mind can be your enemy.
6. Surrender to the flow of the universe.
7. Remember you are not your body or your mind. You are the Witness. You are Spirit.

You will have two assignments this week. Your first is to create your forest. What you will need:
• Poster board
• Magic markers or paints
• Old magazines
• Glue stick

Cut out pictures from a magazine that demonstrate what will bring you happiness in each of the five categories listed above. Do not stop to censor what you believe to be possible, what you believe to be contradictory, or anything that bothers your internal computer. Now, draw five large trees on your poster board and label the bottom of each tree with one of the life categories: 1. career 2. home 3. spouse/partner 4. personal growth and leisure, and 5. family and friends.

Glue the pictures onto each tree and include any motivational words, phrases, or thoughts you feel might be important. When you are finished, share the board with a trusted friend or partner. Hang the poster in a prominent place in your home and allow yourself to feel the joy that your forest promises. Remind yourself often that it is the whole forest that will make you happy and not just climbing one tree.

Climbing Your Pyramid

In order to access our Spirit, which is like powerful and unbound energy, we must follow a five-step process of working through the five layers of our energetic anatomy which we introduced earlier as the koshas. In review, the five koshas are the body, breath, mind, wisdom, and bliss. Working through the five koshas is like climbing the pyramid of life. It's wide at the bottom and filled with our thoughts, aches, and pains, attachments and daily distractions. As we move toward the middle of the pyramid, we start to shed some of the physical baggage. We put less energy into all the external stressors going on around us and begin to focus on our thoughts. We start to see that our mind is its own animal capable of creating our inner reality. To rid ourselves of our incessant thoughts is to, once again, ascend the pyramid. You quickly see that using this metaphor, the higher you can ascend the better and clearer the view. You may even be able to see for miles in all directions. This is the value of one-pointedness. It gives you clarity of vision so that what's below you becomes less important than what's around you in all directions.

If you are interested in climbing your own pyramid of life and reaching one-pointedness, you should start with some activities that nourish your physical body, like yoga, engaging the senses, getting good sleep, eating well, or taking a walk. Once you have found a rhythm with the physical body you can progress to the energy body by doing breathing exercises, acupuncture or reiki, which will help you move prana or chi into your system. You remember from the previous chapter that prana is life-force energy that is present in the universe but sometimes deficient in our bodies. Acupuncture (from a licensed professional) is one of the best ways to feel a renewed sense of spirit and can help heal the body naturally. Oriental Medicine and acupuncture can be used to treat stress, anxiety, depression, pain management, migraines, sleep disorders, cold/flu, and a myriad of other disorders in the body.

Next, move onto your mental body by practicing visualizations, journaling, reading biographies, or engaging in psychotherapy when needed.

Your wisdom body is that place where your conscience resides your intuition or higher mind. Treat it kindly by learning to meditate. Meditation is the cessation of thought and the peace of complete silence in your mind and body. This is one of the more difficult practices and may require a slow start by just sitting quietly for five minutes each day and building stamina slowly, adding time as your mind becomes more disciplined.

Finally, move into your bliss body and begin to see that you are Divine and have the ability to create what you truly want in your life. Tap into this layer of Self through prayer, creating a sacred space, chanting, or learning a sacred mantra.

Meditation

Meditation has been around for thousands of years and stems from Eastern spiritual traditions. Today, it is used both inside and outside its traditional religious and cultural setting for health and wellness purposes. The National Institute for Health (NIH) cites meditation as a practice individuals have used for anxiety, pain, depression, mood, and self-esteem problems, stress, insomnia, and physical or emotional symptoms that may be associated with chronic illness. From this perspective it sounds like it could be a useful tool for the fertility journey, doesn't it?

Although many people are familiar with the concept of meditation, they may be confused by the actual practice or struggle to truly understand its relevance or importance. Perhaps you are among the many who "don't really get it," or wonder if you are doing it right or question what, exactly, is supposed to happen. That's why we would like to take a bit of time in this book to demystify the sacred art of meditation.

Meditation versus Visualization

Let's start out by talking about what meditation is not. Meditation is not hypnosis, auto-suggestion, intense relaxation, a dream or sleep state, an alpha state, or daydreaming. Interestingly, meditation is also not visualization. Visualization is a form of theater of the mind; creating visual images that help bring a person to a state of peace or relaxation. During visualization or guided imagery, the student is generally given oral instructions that engage the five senses or work to progressively relax the body. If you have ever been instructed to imagine yourself on a beautiful white sand beach, breathing fresh air while the rays from the sun gently warm your face, you have probably experienced visualization. Similarly, audio tapes or CDs that tell you to "imagine sperm is meeting egg" or instruct you to progressively relax are also using guided imagery to help take you into deeper states of relaxation or sleep. Visualizations can be extremely useful in the fertility process, particularly if you are the type of person who has a difficult time sitting still or quieting your mind. It is also an excellent primer or foray into the more difficult practice of meditation.

The Meditative Process

So now that you know what meditation is *not*, it is time to discuss what it *is*. Said simply, meditation is the effortless flow of consciousness. It is learning how to suspend the constant chatter of thought that normally occupies the mind in order to achieve a greater sense of physical relaxation, mental clarity, psychological balance, and spiritual connectedness.

It is the process of separating your Witness from your mind and transcending it to the top of the pyramid in order to gain greater insight into the valley below. Through the practice of meditation, one begins to see that the normal state of the mind is unstable, fluctuating from idea to idea, emotional, externally oriented, and influenced by past conditioning. We talked in the Dealing with Disappointment chapter about the affliction of avidya. Avidya, once again, is delusion or mis-knowing; the inability to break free from our own unconscious and erroneous thoughts. Meditation is the process of pulling away from our minds so that we can see how our thinking or past conditioning is incorrect. Meditation helps to de-condition and calm the mind, ultimately leading to discriminating insight and more spontaneous healing.

What Meditation Can Do

Many people who practice meditation use it as a form of prayer to "get things they want." In fact, meditation should be used to get rid of things that are not serving you. What things along your fertility journey could you stand getting rid of in order to make you more fully fertile? How about those negative thoughts or the hatred you feel toward every pregnant woman on the planet? What if you tried to get rid of the desire to control every aspect of the baby-making process? Could life be better for you? These are the types of questions you must ponder for yourself during the course of meditation. Sit quietly and just watch the thoughts begin to bubble up to the surface. Don't judge your thoughts and don't attach yourself to them. Imagine that they are nothing more than big, fluffy clouds floating by your head. You can touch these clouds of thought but don't sit on them or hold on too tight lest they carry you away to the land of the lost. Observing thoughts without participating in their emotional content is a powerful practice that cultivates the calm beneath the storm of our minds.

Research on Meditation

Anecdotal case studies showing the efficacy of meditation on an individual's health date back to the 1950s. It was not until 1961 when B. K. Anand did a study of a yogi in India that meditation started reaching the consciousness of the scientific world. Anand found that his yogi subject could lower his oxygen metabolism at will. There are similar reports of Zen monks in Japan who could also reduce their oxygen consumption by 20 percent during meditation sessions. *(Jevning, 1992)* Through his own studies Herbert Benson, M.D., of the Harvard Medical School and founding president of the Mind/Body Medical Institute, found that Americans who practiced meditation were able to lower their oxygen metabolism an average of 12 percent, an even greater drop than during sleep. A later study of meditation found an even greater 40 percent decline in oxygen consumption and a 50 percent decline in respiration rate. *(Farrow & Herbert, 1982)*

In 1984 Jon Kabat-Zinn authored a very compelling study in which 90 chronic pain patients were trained in meditation in a 10-week stress reduction and relaxation program. The meditation group showed significant reductions in pain, negative body image and inhibition of activity by pain, symptoms, mood disturbance, anxiety, and depression. Usage of drugs for pain management decreased and activity levels and feelings of self-esteem increased. The group that did not use meditation did not show significant improvement on these measures after traditional treatment protocols. It was also determined after follow-up, that the improvements observed during the meditation training were maintained up to 15 months after the training for all measures except present-moment pain. The majority of subjects reported continued high compliance with the meditation practice as part of their daily lives. *(Kabat-Zinn, 1984)*

Today research papers on meditation have shown the practice can lower heart rate, blood pressure and body temperature as well as reduce cortisol (stress-producing hormone) levels. Thyroid-stimulating hormone and growth hormone secretion is also reduced by meditation and levels of arginine vasopressin, thought to play a role in memory and learning, are higher during meditative states. *(O'Halloran, 1985)* Interestingly, serotonin levels were found to increase significantly versus a control group with meditation practice. Serotonin, as you may know, plays a part in the regulation of mood, sleep, learning, and constriction of blood vessels. Low levels of serotonin in the body have been linked to depression. It's great to know that research has now shown the many benefits of meditation on the mind and body which the yogis have known to be true for thousands of years. Research aside, though, the very practical values of meditation for the purposes of your fertility are removal of stress and fear, an improvement in your personality and greater clarity for decision-making. Unfortunately, meditation is one of those things that cannot fully be understood without practice. The benefits deepen with faith in its efficacy and with consistent practice, so let's get started.

By now you have probably already begun to think about your forest and all the things you truly want in life. Now it is time to start ascending your pyramid to see what it is you really want and what it is you think you want. Try one of the following meditiation techniques.

Object of Beauty

Close your eyes and picture in your mind's eye the most beautiful object you have seen or can imagine. This can be man-made, an object in nature, a piece of chocolate cake, whatever. As you sit quietly and breathe, imagine the colors, the shapes, the details and the smells of this object. Engage all of your senses and hold this object in your mind and experience its beauty. When your mind starts thinking about your "to do" list, bring it back to your object of beauty.

Hong Sau

Close your eyes and begin to breathe. In this technique we silently chant "hong" as we inhale and "sau" as we exhale. When the mind wanders, simply bring it back to the breath. Inhaling "hong" and exhaling "sau."

Watching the Breath

Close your eyes and begin to focus on the sun center, the spot on your forehead just above your eyebrows, but mentally watch and listen to the sound of your breath. The sound of the

Preparation for Meditation

- Find a quiet place, away from distraction if possible.
- Sit in a position which allows you to keep your spine straight (in a chair with feet flat on floor, sitting on a cushion on the floor with your back against the wall, or even lying down, although it may be difficult to maintain wakeful awareness in a supine position).
- Begin with a few gentle neck rolls and shoulder shrugs.
- Start with five minutes, building slowly up to longer periods as you are able.

- Work with one technique for a while rather than jumping around from technique to technique.

There are a myriad of meditation techniques available to you. Try one or two of the techniques described above and practice until you feel completely competent with one of them. Once you have a "winner," begin practicing this technique daily.

breath, as you inhale and exhale through the nose, will begin to occupy the mind so you are better able to experience the bliss of pure self-conscious awareness.

E-mantra

Close your eyes and inhale through the nose. As you exhale say the letter "E." Do this for seven or eight rounds and then drop the mantra. Return to E-mantra whenever the mind begins to wander.

Tami writes:

Even after conceiving Kevin and Courtney, my prayers and meditations became all the more important and meaningful. My practice consoled me when I worried that first trimester about whether or not I would be able to carry the babies to term. My meditation practice comforted me each and every day of the 17 weeks I vomited into the toilet. "All for the greater good," I kept telling myself. I remember driving to work one day and noticing, for the first time, that the church on the corner of my street had two very large and stately spires that rose from the building. They stood side by side with a cross on top of each, reaching into the sky above. I remember thinking of those spires as a symbol and object of beauty. Those were my twins growing in my body, strong and sturdy, half way between heaven and earth. By visualizing those spires I was able to connect with my unborn children in a very profound way. They had character and personality, yet they were Divine. Every day I drove past them and every day I used those spires as my object of beauty, my symbolic children. The spires were strong and healthy, just as I prayed my children would be.

I started developing signs of pre-eclampsia around 32 weeks of pregnancy. I was seeing the doctor several times a week and I sensed he was starting to grow concerned. At 34 weeks the right side of my face became paralyzed with Bells Palsy, my ankles were the size of tree trunks, and my arm was tingling with a sudden onset of carpel tunnel.

Some might say that I was in denial at the time about how sick I really was, but I don't think it was denial. It was a knowing deep inside that everything would just be okay. I had ascended the pyramid and was confident enough to know deep inside that, one way or another, the babies would be strong and healthy I focused again on the spires. Looking back, I realize that not only was my daily ritual with the spires a form of meditation, it had become a mantra and affirmation. I was hospitalized at 35 weeks and induced that very same day. I delivered both children vaginally with Kevin weighing six pounds and Courtney four pounds, ten ounces. They had jaundice, but they were okay. No neo-natal intensive care unit, no long hospital stays, no long labor or traumatic birth. My babies were just as I knew they would be: strong and healthy. The spires that had once been my meditative object of beauty that symbolized strength were now manifest in the form of my children.

Prayer

WHEN PDTM OPENED its first brick and mortar center, Dr. Alice Domar came to Chicago to speak at our grand opening. What still stands out as the most interesting element of that talk was Dr. Domar's assertion that most women who have difficulty conceiving experience a crisis of faith on some level. Dr. Domar went on to discuss how her mind/body support groups in Boston grew from being strictly cognitive/behavioral in nature to incorporate discussions of faith and, as Dr. Domar termed it, the "G" word—God. This resonated with our own experience teaching yoga for fertility, where we were finding that the yoga teachings were scratching a spiritual itch in our students.

When you think about it, it makes complete sense that spiritual crisis is a major side effect of infertility. Any woman who sees a pregnant 15-year-old after receiving yet another negative pregnancy result will be hard-pressed not to shake a frustrated fist at the spiritual powers that be. There just seems to be a maddening arbitrariness to who gets pregnant and who doesn't. The painful nature and apparent injustices of infertility can quickly bring issues of sin and punishment to the surface of even the most faithful and leave them feeling bereft of spiritual support.

It could be tempting to give in to this sense of spiritual isolation, but the kosha model we explored in Chapter 9 tells us that this separation from Spirit can also negatively impact both our biological and our psychological fertility. As we learned in chapter 9, the anandamaya kosha, our bliss body, is the spiritual core of our being. If this connection with spirit is absent from our lives, we are working at a fundamental disadvantage. When we restore connection with our bliss body, the healing potential of the kosha model is at its strongest. In other words, when we reaffirm our connection with Spirit, we open a channel of healing that can literally work miracles.

Up until this point in this book, our focus has been on different yogic tools for helping us to create fertility in our physical, mental, and spiritual selves. It is fitting that perhaps the most universal tool in the holistic fertility tool chest is the one we will touch on last—prayer. In this chapter we will discuss our belief in the power of prayer to impact fertility and share with you some of the prayers that guided us and our students while they were trying to conceive.

What is Prayer?

Prayer is an act of communication with a deity or spirit for the purpose of offering praise or gratitude, seeking guidance, or even simply to express thoughts and emotions that burden our hearts. Anthropologists attest that evidence of human prayer dates as far back as 3,000 BCE and that even the most primitive of intelligent human beings practiced something we would today recognize as prayer. There are numerous forms a prayer can take: spontaneous speech, hymns, chants, and incantations are just a few of the ways in which humans pray. And pray they do, still. A 2005 survey conducted by Rasmussen Reports found that 47 percent of Americans pray nearly every day.

In recent years, numerous clinical studies have been conducted to examine the power of prayer but results have been equivocal. In cases where prayer is offered on behalf (intercessory prayer) of patients, both positive and negative associations have been found with length of hospital stay, complications, and other health outcomes. In the case of personal spiritual practice, studies indicate that a spiritual practice may be associated with lower levels of depression in general and improved quality of life during illness, but the relationship is mediated by many confounding factors.

Because many of these studies show potential benefit, prayer and spirituality are gaining attention in the medical community for their potential therapeutic benefits and are considered a Complementary and Alternative Medicine (CAM) technique. In fact, prayer tops the list as the most frequently used CAM technique in the United States.

Yoga, because it is a spiritual practice rather than a religion, does not espouse a belief in any one God or tradition. Instead, yoga uses techniques like asana, breathing, mantra, and meditation to quiet the distractions of body and mind in order to reveal an individual's innate spirituality. However, one of the challenges of yoga for infertility is that many of the more esoteric techniques, such as meditation, are not as easily practiced by beginners in acute situations of pain, loss, and fear. When we're upset, our inner Light appears to be obscured by our troubles. Like a traveler lost in the woods on a stormy night, we have been told the lights of a warm cottage are just up ahead but we can't see them. We're too scared and tired and bereft of hope to believe that warmth and comfort are around the corner so we stop looking for the Light and sit paralyzed in darkness. For such trying times, the yoga tradition recommends that we turn to the practice of prayer to enlist the aid of other great spiritual teachings or Divine Beings in returning us again to our own inner Light.

Navigating Rough Waters

From a yogic perspective, perhaps the most important quality of prayer is its ability to help us recognize and cultivate the qualities of the Divine in our selves, even when the external conditions are stormy. Take for instance this Christmas novena that is often used for fertility in the Catholic Church:

Hail and blessed be the hour and the moment in which the Son of God
was born, of the most pure Virgin Mary at midnight, in Bethlehem, in piercing cold.
In that hour vouchsafe, oh Lord, and hear my prayer and grant my desires
Through the merits of the Lord Jesus Christ and His Blessed Mother,
Amen

This novena is repeated nine times per day (or 12 or 30, depending on which aunt or girlfriend gives you instructions!) in the month leading up to Christmas Day. On the surface it is a simple prayer, but with repetition, the prayer draws attention to the cold, frightening journey of Mary and her family before the birth of Jesus, Mary's courage and patience leading up to that birth and the idea that the Divine birth did not occur under particularly safe or auspicious conditions. Some may find a parallel in this prayer to the challenges of infertility and the idea that sometimes, as the cliché would have it, it's darkest before the dawn. In order to see a rainbow you first have to experience a storm.

There is often also a deep symbolism in prayers. Returning to the Christmas novena, this prayer is offered during Advent, the four weeks leading up to the birth of Jesus in the Christian tradition. This period corresponds to the darkest and shortest days of the year leading up to the winter solstice. As mentioned previously, the winter solstice is celebrated in many cultures as the "return of the light." It is a time for planting the seeds of intention for the coming year. In this context, the novena serves a three-fold purpose. It is a seed of heart-felt intention planted at a time that many spiritual traditions hold to be an important time of new beginnings. It calls upon the image of Mary as an example of courage and it helps us reflect on the connection between our own life and the lives of other, more enlightened beings who have walked paths similar to our own and left us teachings to help us navigate similar rough waters.

Tami writes:

One day, upon learning of my pregnancy with twins, my mother-in-law Carol came bounding through the door, hands filled with what she referred to as her "good luck charms." She handed me a small clay statue of St. Gerard and a few prayer cards of the same. I learned that St. Gerard was the Catholic patron saint of motherhood and child. As the story goes, a young

Gerard was often seen playing with a statue of the Madonna and Child outside the cathedral in his Italian village. He claimed to receive bread from the Madonna every day and faithfully brought it home to his mother. As he grew, the saint had a penchant for the mother and child bond. It is written that he often cured young children of their life-threatening illnesses and saved more than just a few women during their difficult time with childbirth. St. Gerard held special meaning for Carol. She miscarried a child in between the birth of her eldest son, my brother-in-law, and my husband. The miscarriage was late term and devastating to her. She found the prayer of St. Gerard and prayed to it daily that she might conceive another child and carry it to term. She promised that if she was granted this child, she would name him/her after this patron saint of motherhood. Behold my husband, Brian Gerard Quinn, and his younger brother by two years, Paul Gerard Quinn. I was very moved by my mother-in-law's story. I placed the statue on my dresser and winked at him from time to time throughout my pregnancy, acknowledging the bond between him and the Quinn clan. I asked that he bestow upon me whatever sacred energy he held that I, too, might deliver healthy children. My twins were born Kevin Gerard and Courtney Gale.

What if I Don't Believe in God?

So what if you don't believe in God, or never truly connected with a spiritual tradition that feels authentic to you? Can you still pray? Absolutely. If you wish to pray, but are not sure who to pray to, there is a concept in Eastern spiritual tradition that we have found very useful at PDtM. The concept is *"Ishta Devata"*, a practice that invites practitioners to choose a form of divinity that inspires them and to offer prayers to that Source. In this view, the Ishta can be a deity, for instance Jesus or Allah or Krishna, or even a moral concept like "Truth" or "Love," since in all religions these words are synonyms for the Divine.

The concept of the Ishta is based on the idea that many rivers run into the true spiritual Source. Joseph Campbell, author of many books on comparative religion, suggested that the true Source of spirituality is un-nameable and un-knowable, and that all religions are simply an attempt to articulate this force from which everything arose, in which all is currently arising and to which everything will eventually return. Yoga would agree with Campbell's assertion of one Source, but would challenge the notion that the Source of spirit is unknowable. Yoga would suggest that as we turn our attention to prayer and meditation we will eventually meet this Source inside our quieted selves. Line up Krishna, Jesus, Allah, Yaweh, Buddha, and a snow-capped mountain and ask the yogi which one is God and she would answer "They all are, and so am I, because we cannot be separate from the Source." This is not a stance of arrogance or paganism, but an assertion of humble recognition that the Divine is omnipotent and omnipresent and, as such, cannot be separate from human beings. We are a part of life, not apart from it.

Beth writes:

Sometimes you have to walk before you can run. Tami and I still laugh about our first foray into teaching the concept Ishta Devata in our PDtM Fertility Yoga classes. On the last night of our very first PDtM yoga class, we decided to close the session with an Ishta Devata visualization. This practice instructs students to visualize their Ishta Devata, or "personal deity," and to draw this Divine source into their hearts to help them in their fertility journey. Okay, it was an ambitious exercise for a group of yoga newbies. We know that now. At the time we were simply bubbling over with the desire to teach as much yoga as we could while we had these folks in class.

After the class Matt and I had dinner with our friends Marty and Elise, who were in the throes of IVF and taking part in the class as students. When Marty, whose own faith is agnostic, began to relate his experience of the Ishta meditation, I saw that we'd overshot our mark.

"When Tami said I should visualize a Being or symbol that represents my spiritual source, the only thing that came to my mind was Elise (his wife). Then I thought that was weird because, you know, Elise is my wife, not my Ishta. So I erased that and the next thing that popped into my mind was our dogs Nagi and Gidget. Then I started to panic because that was totally wrong and ended up with an Ishta that had Gidget's body with Elise's head!"

"It was the word 'symbol' that got me," Elise added. "Once I heard that the only thing I could visualize was a big, yellow, 'have a nice day' smiley face!"

Clearly, Marty and Elise's honest (and hilarious) feedback drove home the point that for many of us who are not steeped in a religious practice, the concept of Ishta Devata isn't an easy one.

Truth be told, even my own experience of this meditation took time to build—I spent a lot of time trying to get rid of Elise's vision of the smiley face! For a while the Ishta was a revolving door of images from my childhood Catholicism as I tried on different saints and biblical folk until finally, in one deep effort, I saw a vision of the pieta, Mary the Mother holding the dead body of her Son. Once I saw this image in my mind, tears sprung to my eyes and I felt an instant sense of connection shoot down into my heart. Having just experienced the death of a child through a still birth, I related to Mary as a mother, and to the grief she must have felt at losing a child, to her strength in going on beyond loss with her faith in God intact. Her powerful image bolstered my strength as I went on to try again to conceive after my loss and I would pray to her often during my deepest bouts of grief. Because the qualities of the pieta resonated so deeply in my life at that time, I felt inspired by praying to this symbol of courage. Far more than being words that came from my mouth, I knew my prayers flowed directly from my heart and kindled in me the courage I needed to try to get pregnant again.

In the years since that first exploration of my Ishta, it has changed several times. As I struggle to balance work and parenting I find myself turning often to the Buddha's middle

Prayers to St. Gerard

Feast Day: October 16

For Motherhood:
O good St. Gerard, powerful intercessor before the throne of God, wonder-worker of our day, I call upon you and seek your help. While on earth, you always fulfilled God's designs; help me, too, to always do God's holy will. Beseech the master of life, from whom all parenthood proceeds, to bless me with offspring, that I may raise up children to God in this life and heirs to the kingdom of God's glory in the life to come.
Amen.

For Mother With Child:
O almighty and everlasting God, through the Holy Spirit, you prepared the body and soul of the glorious virgin Mary to be a worthy dwelling place of your divine Son. Through the same Holy Spirit, you sanctified St. John the Baptist, while still in his mother's womb. Hear the prayers of your humble servant who implores you, through the intercession of St. Gerard, to protect me amid the dangers of childbearing and to watch over the child with which you blessed me. May this child be cleansed by the saving water of baptism and, after a Christian life on earth, may we, both mother and child, attain everlasting bliss in heaven.
Amen.

way. When I am in a particularly angry and judgmental state of mind or crabby with my children, I might pray to Jesus for the ability to forgive and let go of my negative thoughts and emotions. In times of joy and gratitude I might offer thanks to Lakshmi, the Hindu goddess of surplus and prosperity. For some my spiritual habits may seem fickle, or even sacrilegious. I do not think this is so. In my eyes, each Ishta is a gift from God that reveals another facet of a power that is far, far beyond the grasp of my human understanding. And they make me feel closer to the Light that I know shines at the core of my being.

Make It Personal

As Beth's story reveals, our Ishta should resonate with our body, mind and spirit. Like the image of the pieta described previously, when an Ishta reflects traits we value or are missing in ourselves or wish to cultivate in our lives, reverence to this being or ideal takes on an authenticity and intimacy. Since another goal of prayer is to cultivate and reveal the qualities of the Divine in ourselves, it helps if we choose an Ishta that is personally inspiring. Most traditions offer saints, elders, and sages that have different symbolic roles, so if you feel more comfortable, you may wish to stay within the context of a spiritual tradition that is comfortable and familiar to you. If you are currently re-exploring the concept of Spirit and wish to open to a broader spectrum of Ishtas, you can take this opportunity to broaden your knowledge of other spiritual traditions to see if you find one that lights your heart.

This next exercise will help you explore the kinds of qualities you revere and desire to bring into your life and will help point the way to possible Ishtas.

WEEK 12 ACTIVITY 1: FINDING YOUR ISHTA

Take a sheet of paper and place three headings at the top: heart, mind, and spirit. Under these headings begin to list first the qualities you admire about yourself in each of these areas and then the qualities you would like to cultivate in these areas. Don't worry if you come across contradictions; humans are complicated. Just keep writing.

Once you have finished, look for themes or qualities that are present in all three categories. For instance, if under heart you wrote "good friend" as something you like, under mind you wrote "compassionate," and under spirit you wrote "need to belong" you might find that your Ishta could be a Buddha of compassion like the Buddha, Jesus Christ, or Krishna. Feel free to range wide and explore different spiritual traditions. Remember also that concepts such as Truth and Love can also become the recipient of your prayer. If you choose a concept, you can take the process one step further by meditating on the concept to see if it reveals a symbol. If you wanted to pray for Fertility, to choose one relevant example, your meditation might reveal archetypical images of fertility such as a flower, the moon, or a field of grain. While it may seem strange to offer prayers to a flower, remember that the flower is a symbol of the Divine quality of fertility.

Beginning to Pray

Why Do It?

The idea of God in mysticism is pure internal consciousness, but there is no power in consciousness so we need a symbol that is external to ourselves. We need a symbol that is our "not-self." We need to get our energy to attune to our higher consciousness because we become that which we attune to. That is the value of prayer. Whatever you think you need is exactly what you need and when you attune to your highest Self, you become your highest Self.

Tami writes:

One of the most common requests I receive at PDtM as a yoga teacher and Swami is, "I'm beginning to think prayer would benefit my conception journey. I'm not very religious so what can I do to connect with God?"

When we are experiencing fertility trouble or any life challenges, we need a shoulder to lean on and a dumping ground for getting rid of all the garbage that goes along with those challenges. In my discussions with students about why praying is difficult for them, there are three reasons consistently cited:

1. We have become increasingly skeptical of religion as we see how, in recent years, it has sparked war and division in the world rather than peace and unity. Instead of turning to the roots of our religious upbringing during times of personal crisis, we turn away in search of something more fulfilling or more relevant for our life situation. We get the idea that the old way "just doesn't work anymore" and feel challenged to go beyond the scope of what is familiar. We rightfully try seeking that which is spiritual rather than that which is religious and often become lost in our search, not knowing where to turn or whom to ask for help. Perhaps this is why there is curiosity about some of the newer practices like Scientology or renewed interest in older, more mystical faiths like Cabbalism. Through our desire to land in an appropriate spiritual house, we entertain ideas and concepts we might never have dreamed of before.

2. The world is becoming more and more secular. There is greater tolerance for inter-faith marrying which means families are becoming more heterogeneous in their religious practices. When Christian mom marries Jewish dad one of three things usually happens: they become a blended family celebrating both traditions, they choose not to celebrate either in an attempt to avoid conflict, or the family chooses one faith for the entire household. Confusion for the children can result when the parents do not make a commitment to teaching them the prayers, tenets, or rituals for a particular faith. Rather than choose one parent's faith over another's, the children are often left feeling a bit non-committal as they try to adopt or form their own religious convictions into adulthood.

3. Some folks have just never learned how to pray or do not know to whom they are praying. This state of purgatory is okay as long as life is shaping up just the way you want it. When presented with challenges or crisis, however, it is easy to understand how connecting with something bigger than your problems can be therapeutic. There are, after all, some issues that only God or a higher power can solve.

Although we have come a long way in having greater tolerance for religious differences, one thing seems to be getting lost along the way and that's our sense of ritual and tradition. These things are often perceived as "old-fashioned" or too dogmatic for modern-day acceptance.

The trouble is we still really need them. When trying to have a baby, we need things like clearing ceremonies, loss rituals, meditation, and prayer to truly help us heal our spiritual anatomy. That is why we have included a number of ritualistic or prayerful exercises in this book. It gets you connected with God, your higher power, Divine energy or whatever euphemism you choose to call it and that's all a part of becoming Fully Fertile. So when those students present to me their challenges in praying, I suggest they find their Ishta, because it's a direct phone line to pure consciousness.

Prayer Through Surrender

If you're rusty, one of the easiest places to get back in the swing of prayer is during the rest period at the end of your yoga posture practice. As you recall from the first chapter of the book, after our physical practice, we always take time to rest in Svasana, or corpse pose. In addition to providing deep physical relaxation and a chance for the work of practice to become integrated both neurologically and energetically, Svasana is an act of symbolic (and eventually active) surrender. The word Svasana actually means corpse pose, and traditional yogis would often accompany Svasana with a graphic meditation of the death and decomposition of the physical body. While that practice has fallen from vogue for obvious reasons, Svasana is still a wonderful place to practice the "death of ego" and invite powers beyond ourselves to take up the reigns and steer the ship for a bit. As we let go of our self with a little "s," we invite in the qualities of Self with a big one. All that is necessary to make Svasana an act of prayer is to lie down with the intention of allowing the qualities of Spirit to fill and nourish you. You will be amazed at the effect of this simple practice.

One student, Eloise, attributed the practice of Svasana to her ability to make the shift to donor gametes. Eloise's case was an interesting one. Her marriage was both her and her husband's second, and both brought biological children to the new union. Her husband had a vasectomy reversal which failed to produce viable sperm. The idea of moving to donor sperm was initially difficult for Eloise, because she wanted to cement this new marriage with a child that would share their genetics. Although she and her husband eventually became comfortable with the idea of donor sperm, multiple failed IVFs with donor sperm suggested Eloise might have fertility issues also; in fact her FSH was slightly high. Nevertheless, she continued with IUIs.

The process stretched on until nearly two years had elapsed without a pregnancy. In one emotional yoga session, we discussed whether Eloise actually wanted a child or whether she wanted to prove to herself she could have another one. She recognized that her odds of conception using both donor egg and sperm were the quickest route to a baby.

After our physical practice ended, we took Svasana. Eloise brought a deep affinity with the earth religions and shamanistic practices of Central America to her yoga practice. After one particular practice she entered Svasana with the intention of hearing the voice of Mother Earth. When Svasana ended she came back from deep relaxation with clarity that the route of donor egg/sperm was part of her overall work of celebrating her new, blended family. Eloise entered the donor gamete process shortly after this revelation and now she's the mother of an amazing six-month-old girl named Jillian. If you ask Eloise and her husband which baby they were supposed to create, Jillian or another "biological" child, they both laugh and ask their baby the same question. Jillian just beams back into their adoring eyes.

Other Forms of Prayer

Apart from the simple act of surrender described above, there are many other ways to pray. In the next section we will briefly touch on some of these methods.

Jeanie's prayer:

I went to a church for the first time as a sophomore in college. Since I had never prayed in the Christian tradition before, I did not know how to do it. I remember thinking of it like writing a letter to Santa: "Dear God, please let me get what I want...Amen." As a small girl, I remember praying to have blond hair and blue eyes, like most of my friends. But I am not sure if prayer is really supposed to be used to help us get what we want.

I was raised in Buddhism where chanting is commonly used to help people get in touch with the natural flow of the universe. We also pray, but I think that both of these practices aim for the same goal: recognizing our connectedness to the whole. I still feel like a novice in terms of praying (in the Western sense). But I know that I do have faith in the universe and that our intention plays a great role in the direction of our future. It can be helpful to pray for the things you want; action follows intention, but it can also be helpful to pray for non-material things like peace and acceptance.

As we mentioned before in discussing the negative impact of stress, developing your acceptance and working on your attitude is just as important as working on your body. Don't just pray for the things you cannot control (I still have black hair and brown eyes, like all Koreans); pray for the ability to relinquish the need for control. Pray for understanding and enlightenment. With this, your energy will flow more freely and this will help you be in a better place to conceive.

In Oriental Medicine, it is understood that the Heart houses the Spirit and is intimately tied with emotions. It is said that meditation and praying can empty our minds and clear our hearts so that our soul can reside peacefully there.

Pray that you can realize your full potential.

And I pray for all of you, who read this book, that you may find balance in your lives and serenity in your hearts. May you all become Fully Fertile.

Verbal Prayer

Verbal prayer can either be spontaneous, whereupon the individual offering the prayer simply speaks her mind to the Spiritual Source, or traditional, where existing prayers like the example of the Christmas novena are used. Both methods of prayer are useful. The first allows for an unprecedented freedom of expression and an unburdening of the heart. It is through spontaneous prayer that we can often ask for forgiveness or guidance for a particular issue or challenge in our lives. Traditional prayer carries other benefits. First, if grief is too strong or it is too difficult to express a complexity of emotion, the repetition of "well worn words" of traditional prayer can often bring about peace of mind.

Almost all spiritual traditions extend verbal prayer to include the practice of chanting. The word chant comes from the Latin for "sing" and chanting is the hymn-like repetition of sacred verses including psalms, mantras, or prayers. In other words, chanting gives sacred texts a rhythm and sometimes a melody that aids us in repetition. In yoga this practice of chanting is called "kirtan", originally a Sikh tradition where sacred mantras were chanted to classical Indian ragas or melodies. With the growing popularity of yoga, kirtan has grown to include modern musical instruments, even electric guitar. Prayer can also take the form of singing hymns. At Midnight Mass our pastor used to joke that the choir got a double dip at the prayer fountain and promised that if we sang really loud for every hymn it would be like praying twice!

If verbal prayer or singing hymns isn't part of your current regimen, try experimenting with CDs of different hymns—gospel, classical or modern kirtan, the chanting of Buddhist or Gregorian monks—in your car. The musical element of hymns or chants can create a healing vibration that is remarkably uplifting. You may find yourself belting out "This Little Light of Mine" on your way to work or chanting "Om Namah Shivaya" on your way home.

The Lifespan of a Fertility Yoga Practice. Beth writes:

One of my yoga teachers said that practicing yoga is like a crash course in reincarnation. In one yoga practice you're a dog, a tree, and an eagle, and then a warrior, and in another you're a pigeon, then a shape like a triangle, and then a cobra...until sooner or later you've been transformed into so many different things you start to recognize the "One in the all and the All in the one." I have always loved this idea because it moves asana practice beyond just physical stretching and strengthening and illustrates a basic tenet of practice: yoga asana is transformative beyond the physical body. In each posture there is a wisdom that becomes imprinted in your being and that wisdom will reveal itself in different ways.

As I mentioned in the introduction to this section of the book, I began my yoga practice at the same time that I embarked on my fertility journey. In my earliest days of yoga I was absolutely fascinated by the physical postures. I would practice eagle pose (see page 54) and try to "feel" the eagle. Whenever I would see a dog stretching his shoulders like we do in downward dog (see page 148), I would smile at him in recognition. As my desire to get pregnant grew, I would work with each posture and ask it what sort of wisdom it could offer me on my quest to conceive. Early on I realized that deep hip openers like pigeon helped to reduce tension in my low back and increase my hip mobility. Twists and folds helped to improve my digestion. Eagle pose was a wonderful detoxifier of stagnant tissues. When I became pregnant for the first time I was so very grateful to the magic of these poses and the wisdom that helped to heal my body.

But, as we know, my journey wasn't going to be an easy one. I had a miscarriage shortly after my first positive pregnancy test. After the loss, when I went back to my yoga practice, I found that I came with a slightly different focus. While I was still looking to the postures for healing and physical benefit, I was much more cognizant of their emotional effects. The grief from the miscarriage had lingered much longer than I expected it would. I especially found that back bends allowed me to let sadness and depression flow through me instead of being bottled up and suppressed. Another of my teachers recommended that I use my yoga to cry every last tear I had inside and that's what I did. I went back to my trees, eagles, and dogs and cried in each, sometimes without knowing why I was crying. And when I realized that the pain of the miscarriage was finally leaving me, I recognized that the yoga poses had healed my emotions and mind as effectively as they had healed my body.

Certain poses were more straightforward in revealing their benefits than others, but the most interesting by far of all asana "wisdom" came through my practice of Sirsasana, or headstand pose. Now don't get me wrong…it's a wonderful posture—very challenging—but

Thoughts in Solitude

We have some favorite prayers and chants that have helped us over the years at PDtM. This one by Sir Thomas Merton is a wonderful prayer for those in crisis. Its humble stance and affirmation of faith can help in dark times.

My Lord God, I have no idea where I am going. I do not see the road ahead of me. I cannot know for certain where it will end. Nor do I really know myself, and the fact that I think I am following Your will does not mean that I am actually doing so. But I believe that the desire to please You does in fact please You. And I hope I have that desire in all that I am doing. I hope that I will never do anything apart from that desire. And I know that, if I do this, You will lead me by the right road, though I may know nothing about it. Therefore I will trust You always though I may seem to be lost and in the shadow of death. I will not fear, for You are ever with me, and You will never leave me to face my perils alone.

SIR THOMAS MERTON

one that always struck me as, I don't know…frivolous. In standing on my head I wasn't stretching my hamstrings, it wasn't too terribly strenuous or requiring of strength, nor was it particularly calming. It took a lot of concentration, certainly, but I wasn't really sure what it was doing. In some ways it felt silly or show-off-ish. Like I was standing on my head just because I could!

Nevertheless, I practiced headstands regularly and learned to become more peaceful in such a challenging pose. But what was this pose going to teach me? I wondered and wondered. But soon I had to stop standing on my head because (hallelujah!) I was pregnant again!

Of course I was nervous, having tried so hard and miscarrying during my last go-round. But there was no cause for concern. I had a lovely but nauseating first trimester, a radiant second trimester, and anticipatory third trimester, and then…

A stillbirth at 38 weeks. A perfect little girl that we named Georgia.

There are still no words I have courage enough to write that could describe the utter shock of losing a healthy baby two weeks before she was due to arrive. I can only say that it was something that I will never, ever forget. It changed my life forever. In that moment I realized the gift of Sirsasana. The moment I learned that Georgia had died, everything I was expecting—baby, joy, family, laughter, amazement—was erased. In that moment my entire life turned upside down. Upside down. My entire life turned upside down.

In the days that followed the loss, I returned to the mat. My body was very beaten up from the rigors of childbirth minus the prize at the end. I was so, so very sad, too. I can remember my first yoga practice after Georgia died. My husband and I went to our mats in our yoga room and began to breathe. Within moments I was crying and suddenly I felt at a complete loss. In all my previous yoga practices I had come with one intention: let me get pregnant. Even after the miscarriage I had practiced with the desire to get pregnant again. But somehow, this evening, the words just stuck in my spiritual throat.

So I just began to practice. Without request, without desire—simply practice. Matt and I went through all of our favorite postures and cried as we did. At the end of practice, we took headstand. Having been pregnant, it was months since my last Sirsasana. I was wobbly and timid as I pressed my legs up to the sky.

And then I heard a voice (again with the voices!) saying "Let go of your expectations, Beth, just let go." And I answered back, "Okay, how?"

How?

The gifts of Sirsasana had finally shown themselves. One of the first things we learn in headstand is how to orient ourselves when our surroundings change. Where are my feet? Well, they're above my head. That's not where they're supposed to be but at least I know where they are. What does the world look like? Okay, it's upside down but at least I know that *and I can begin to look around and get my bearings. My baby was not "supposed" to have died. But she did. I was supposed to be immersed in bliss, not grief. My husband and I were supposed to be parents…not trying to conceive again. And I knew that Matt and I were meant to be parents so that meant I had to eventually think about "trying" again. And my yoga practice changed yet again after this experience. Rather than physical benefit or emotional balancing, my practice became my prayer. I began to ask the universe for guidance each time I stepped on my mat.*

"Guide my steps, reveal my path, and give me strength to walk with an open heart, free of fear. In this way I will be a force of good in this world," became my mantra, or prayer, as I practiced. Weeks passed and the prayer remained the same. Please just let the peace and truth of this practice guide my steps.

Amazingly, it was this prayer that brought the most profound shift of all in my fertility. Shortly after beginning this "new" practice I met Tami and we started the class that became PDtM. Through PDtM I received the opportunity to sow the wonderful seeds of yoga teachings in the open hearts of women, who like me, were seeking a child. Everything had shifted once I opened my definition of fertility beyond the physical. I am not at all surprised that it was not long after starting PDtM that I conceived and finally delivered my son, Jackson, or that when it came time to "try again" my son Calvin was conceived the first time we "tried."

Teaching yoga at PDtM over the years has also made me realize that fertility is not simply biological. So many women have found that alternative forms of family building (using donor gametes, gestational surrogates, adoption) resonate deeply with their own paths in life. There's often a process of letting go of expectations, plans, and schedules (which is what the entire second section of this book is about) as well as a welcoming of what is and what can be. Yoga at its deepest level allows us to open to the possibility of each moment as it arises, be present without judgment, and keep an open mind about the future. It took a while for me to realize this, but all along yoga kept whispering to me that if I did the practice…

All is coming.

So now we've told you our fertility stories and shared with you the wisdom yoga shared with us along the way. Now it's your turn—so what's your fertility story? The last page of this book has been left blank for you to record the story of the family you're meant to have…

Know that our prayers are with you. Namaste,

- Beth, Tami, and Jeanie

My Fertility Story

APPENDIX A: Help Along the Way: Finding a Holistic Practitioner

After reading this book, you may wonder how to find the practitioners or holistic services which are best for you. Interestingly, it is our experience that once you locate one key fertility practitioner, she or he will likely guide you in the direction of other holistic fertility specialists. You may be hard-pressed to find someone in your area who has been specifically trained in or is knowledgeable about fertility. The onus is on you. Beware of general practitioners who claim to also have specialties in treating fertility. While many do, and are extremely gifted practitioners, others may think or wish they do. The first step is to do a bit of research. Ask friends, family members, or other women you know who have used holistic treatments in their fertility journey. Once you have a recommendation, don't just call and book an appointment. It's a wise idea to interview them before your initial session.

Finding an Acupuncturist

Oriental Medical school is a three- to four-year Master's degree program which focuses on both Eastern and Western medical theory and practice. All graduates must pass a state or national board exam before they may be licensed. Each state has its own requirements for licensure so you should look into your own state's Department of Professional Regulations. The National Certification Commission for Acupuncture and Oriental Medicine (NCCAOM) is a certification board and a governing body that administers the national board exam and grants certification to qualified applicants. Most states require and rely on NCCAOM certification as a criterion for the state licensure. The website *www.nccaom.org* lists qualified practitioners in your area.

Questions for Practitioners

Here are some guidelines we suggest you keep in mind as you interview potential practitioners.

- What percentage of your practice is fertility?
- Tell me what you know about fertility medications, ART procedures and any potential contraindications/benefits of combining your modality with my fertility treatment. It is easy for someone to say "Sure, I know all about treating fertility," but we suggest you seek concrete proof that this practitioner has studied, read, and practiced in a significant, real-life way.
- If you are seeing an acupuncturist or yoga teacher already who does not know whether or not something is appropriate for you, err on the side of caution or find a different practitioner.

Don't be shy about asking a lot of questions. We recommend that you speak with several practitioners and ask them about their experience in treating cases like yours. While most practitioners who have been through an accredited OM program will be able to help you, those with more experience regarding fertility (both Eastern and Western) will be able to help you more.

Other Healing Practices

In addition to nutrition, yoga and OM, there are several other techniques we recommend at PDtM. These include fertility massage and Mayan abdominal work, reiki, and astrology. Read on for a brief description of these treatments.

Fertility Massage

Fertility massage is a process of learning where we as individuals hold our stress and tension, and it can be a valuable tool in becoming fully fertile. Practical benefits of massage therapy may include detoxification of body tissues, decreased stress response, improvements in sleep and digestion, and increased overall well-being. We're often asked what makes a massage a fertility massage. That's the question you need to ask your massage therapist. Don't despair if the massage therapist doesn't specialize in fertility massage—a regular old Swedish can do wonders for reducing stress and increasing blood flow. If a practitioner is suggesting fancy techniques, abdominal work, pressure points, or aromatherapy specific for fertility, make sure he or she is well versed in the process of trying to conceive and can assure you that all techniques are appropriate for where you are in your reproductive cycle.

Mayan Abdominal Massage (MAM)

Mayan abdominal massage is a non-invasive external abdominal technique to guide and reposition the internal abdominal organs for optimal health. It is believed in Mayan tradition that in a woman, the uterus represents the center. If the uterus is out of balance, so are the physical, emotional, and spiritual aspects of a woman. In women, these imbalances can manifest as menstrual irregularities, fibroids, endometriosis, polyps, headaches, depression, bladder infections, painful intercourse, irregular bowel movements, and infertility. The imbalance of the uterus can be caused by traumatic injury or surgery in the abdominal area, previous pregnancies and miscarriages, strenuous exercises, time and gravity, and history of physical or mental abuse.

During the MAM session, the practitioner will ask the patient to complete an extensive patient history form. The imbalances are diagnosed and discussed before the practitioner begins to perform MAM that runs about 1 to 2 hours. Upon completion of the MAM, the practitioner will teach the patient how to do self-care techniques at home to increase the efficacy of the MAM session. Depending on the imbalance of the patient, the practitioner may also recommend herbal remedies, castor oil packs and lifestyle and nutritional adjustments. To find a MAM practitioner, please visit the website *www.arvigomassage.com*.

Reiki

The word "Reiki" in Japanese is a combination of two characters that represent Spirit and Energy. In reiki the practitioner acts as a conduit for bringing universal life-force energy (prana or chi) into the body of the recipient. In addition, a gifted reiki practitioner can help balance your energetic anatomy and chakras, and may have insights into some of the ways in which prana is being blocked or drained from your system. While you may not expect it, reiki can be very relaxing and cathartic. This is one treatment we recommend you try.

Aromatherapy

You may recognize that certain smells—the smoke from a chimney on an early autumn night, the smell of lilacs or fresh-mown grass—can trigger an immediate emotional and physical response, often linked to long-term memories of childhood. This is because olfaction, our sense of smell, is closely linked to the limbic system, a primitive part of our brain that mediates the responses of our "fight or flight" chemicals and our endocrine system. The limbic system is also related to the formation of long-term memory. Because of the power and immediacy of our response to different smells, scent-therapy is a wonderful addition to your box of stress-reducing tools.

We use three kinds of aromatherapy at PDtM: incense (mostly used for rituals and ceremonies), essential oils, and flower essences that have been blended with essential oils. Make sure the aroma products you choose are natural, organic, and therapeutic-grade. Any aroma candles you burn should be soy-based rather than paraffin wax-based. Paraffin contains pollutants and toxins that can be harmful to our health and reproduction.

What is a Flower Essence?

A flower essence is the life vibration of a wild flower distilled into oral drops or a spray. They are used in many holistic healing sciences and shamanic traditions. According to these teachings, each species of wildflower holds a particular energetic imprint and healing quality. The essences are used to treat emotional and physical imbalance.

There are several different ways to use a flower essence spray. By spritzing after a yoga practice, we can dispel mental and emotional toxins that linger in our personal energy field. These sprays are also a nice addition to the start of meditation or breathing practice, to break off negative thought patterns and to help settle and ground our attention in the moment.

Astrology

The ancients established that there seems to be a connection between the evolving positions of the planets to a woman's astrological chart and when she is truly fertile. This is especially evident in the relationship of the moon: a woman's fertile capacity is connected to the phase of the moon at the time of her own birth. Understanding the phases of the moon can offer additional help to those who want to pinpoint the most fertile time to start an ART cycle or to conceive naturally.

For more information on astrology and fertility cycles, please visit PDtM's website at *www.pullingdownthemoon.com*.

APPENDIX B: Menstrual Cycle and Basal Body Temperature

The Menstrual Cycle

The menstrual cycle is a complex interweaving of many different cycles in a woman's body. The greater menstrual cycle can be broken down into smaller organ cycles and phases. There is the ovarian cycle, where the follicles develop and ovulate according to the hormonal changes in the ovaries. While this happens, there is also the uterine cycle, where endometrial tissue is built up and sloughed off in the uterus, again, in response to the changes in hormones. The menstrual cycle involves many organs, biorhythms, substances, and glands. A problem with any of these constituent systems can result in impaired fertility.

What is known as the average menstrual period is 28 to 30 days from the beginning of one menstrual period to the next. However, every woman has her own regularity (or irregularity) and may not follow an exact 28- to 30-day cycle, with ovulation on day 14. It is important to try and learn what's normal for you so you can better predict ovulation. Let's look at the menstrual cycle in more detail day by day.

DAYS 1 TO 5

The first phase of the cycle is the menstruation. If a woman is pregnant, the body will create progesterone to support fetal development. When there is no implantation, the progesterone and estrogen levels drop, signaling the body to shed the endometrial lining and begin developing new follicles for ovulation. Average length of menstrual bleeding can be from 2 to 7 days and the amount of menstrual bleeding can vary. In OM, we learn a lot from the menstrual bleeding. Pay attention to the amount and color of menstrual blood, presence of clots, and pain before, during, or after.

DAYS 5 TO 13

In the ovaries, FSH, also known as follicle-stimulating hormone, triggers the follicles to develop. In a given cycle, a group of follicles are developed, only the best candidate being selected to mature and ovulate. The developing follicles produce and release estrogen. This estrogen then stimulates release of more FSH (from hypothalamus and pituitary gland) and causes the uterine lining (endometrium) to thicken. The thickened uterine lining is necessary for nourishing and supporting fetal growth. The rise in estrogen will also stimulate the cervical environment to become more basic (less acidic), as it is normally very acidic. This helps the sperm to survive longer in the cervical environment. This is one reason why the timing of intercourse is very important.

DAY 14

When the dominant follicle nears maturity, luteinizing hormone (LH), produced by the hypothalamus and pituitary gland, will cause the egg to be released from the follicle. The egg is released into the pelvic cavity and is picked up by the fallopian tube. Fertilization occurs in the fallopian tube.

With the sperm present, fertilization can occur about six hours after ovulation. It can take many hours for sperm to reach the egg, therefore, it is good practice to start having intercourse before ovulation. Once the embryo is fertilized, it travels through the fallopian tube to the uterus.

During this journey, the embryo goes through many cell divisions to develop and prepare for implantation in the uterus. The time it takes from the fertilization in the fallopian tube to the implantation in the uterus is about seven days.

THE MENSTRUAL CYCLE

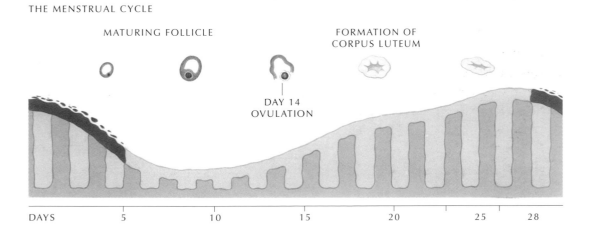

MATURING FOLLICLE   FORMATION OF
                                     CORPUS LUTEUM

DAY 14
OVULATION

DAYS   5   10   15   20   25   28

Many women believe that having intercourse every day during ovulation is the quickest route to conception. We'll discuss this more fully when we get to the bedroom section, but suffice it to say that we do not need to have intercourse every day during this fertile period in order for conception to take place. In fact, some specialists recommend the every-other-day approach during the fertile period in order to allow your partner's sperm to replenish.

DAYS 15 TO 28
In the ovary, after ovulation occurs, the left-over follicle turns into what is called the corpus luteum and begins to secrete progesterone. The secretion of progesterone from the corpus luteum will further thicken the uterine lining into a sponge-like layer with more blood supply, ready to support implantation. The corpus luteum has a finite number of days, usually 14 days after ovulation. If implantation occurs, the corpus luteum lives on and secretes progesterone to support pregnancy. If no implantation occurs, the uterine lining is sloughed off and the cycle begins again.

Charting BBT

One of the best ways to understand your menstrual cycle is to keep a record of your Basal Body Temperature (BBT), or waking body temperature. Normal body temperature is 98.6°F or 37°C . It is noted that a woman's body temperature rises about 0.4–0.5°F after ovulation, which causes the BBT chart to have the biphasic pattern.

Charting basal body temperature is one of the cheapest, and if done correctly, most effective ways to predict ovulation. The only tools that you need are a BBT chart (see Table A1.1, or many fertility websites have BBT charts to download), a thermometer (digital thermometers are much easier to work with than the mercury ones) and an unbroken, good night's sleep for three to five hours. Take your temperature orally, first thing in the morning before getting out of bed, and be as consistent as possible about the time you take it. BBT thermometers are available and they can be more sensitive; but any thermometer will do.

Along with taking BBT, it is helpful to note changes that may happen with the menstrual cycle: such as cervical mucus secretion, changes in the breasts, emotional changes, headaches, and any abnormal bleeding during the cycle. All of this information can give you clues to understanding the body better. Especially from the perspective of OM, the menstrual cycle is a barometer of a woman's inner balance.

Keep both the thermometer and the chart on your nightstand and take the temperature first thing in the morning before anything else.

Guidelines for Charting BBT

- *Make sure to have the BBT chart, a pen or a pencil, and a digital thermometer on your nightstand so that you can take the temperature first thing in the morning.*
- *Day 1 of the cycle is the day that you start your period. If you miss day 1, start from day 2 and chart it as day 2.*
- *Charting time should be consistent each day, within half an hour. Inconsistency in waking time will result in inconsistency in waking temperature. This will limit the usefulness of the chart.*
- *Do not forget to plot the temperature on the BBT.*
- *Record any changes in the body as mentioned previously: e.g. mid-cycle bleeding, breast tenderness, cervical mucus secretion, headaches, cramps, facial breakouts, changes in bowel habits, etc.*
- *Some people will have a drop in BBT just before ovulation. This could help couples to better time when to have intercourse.*
- *Luteal phase, the phase after ovulation, should have a temperature slightly higher than the follicular phase of about 0.4 to 0.5°F.*
- *Don't worry if your chart is not a textbook example. Very few people have a picture perfect BBT chart.*
- *Chart for at least three menstrual cycles to see any changes in pattern of the BBT.*

This tends to be most inconvenient during the weekends, when you want to sleep in later. Tracking BBT may be a bit of a pain but a few months of careful charting can tell you volumes about your cycles. Please do your best in this record keeping. If you're seeing an acupuncturist, he or she can use your chart as another tool to formulate the optimal treatment plan for you.

TABLE A1.1 BBT CHART

Day	1	2	3	4	5	6	7	8	9	10	11	12	13	14	15	16	17	18	19	20	21	22	23	24	25	26	27	28	29	30	31	32	33	34	35	36	37	38	39	40
Date																																								
Time Temp taken																																								
99.7F																																								
99.6																																								
99.5																																								
99.4																																								
99.3																																								
99.2																																								
99.1																																								
99.0																																								
98.9																																								
98.8																																								
98.7																																								
98.5																																								
98.5																																								
98.4																																								
98.3																																								
98.2																																								
98.1																																								
98.0																																								
97.9																																								
97.8																																								
97.7																																								
97.6																																								
97.5																																								
Intercourse																																								
Cervical Mucus																																								
Bleeding spotting																																								
Cramps																																								
Bloating																																								
Breast Tenderness																																								
Others																																								

APPENDIX C: Male and Female Anatomy

MALE REPRODUCTIVE ANATOMY AND PHYSIOLOGY

An entire book could be written about men and their fertility issues. Semen analysis should be the first test a couple undergoes when they suspect infertility. The test is simple, painless, and there are even over-the-counter testing products that couples can use in the privacy of their own home. If sperm count looks good, a woman should proceed with the more invasive, time-consuming, and expensive testing for female fertility issues. You may be surprised to learn that 30–40 percent of the time, a male fertility issue is contributing to a couple's difficulty in conceiving. Causes of male infertility include poor sperm quality or quantity, varicoceles, depletion of testosterone, impotence, cancer treatment, and the inability to reverse a vasectomy, to name a few. Your urologist, reproductive endocrinologist, and holistic practitioners have many techniques to help you get your "swimmers" back in the race. The following section briefly outlines male reproductive anatomy and function.

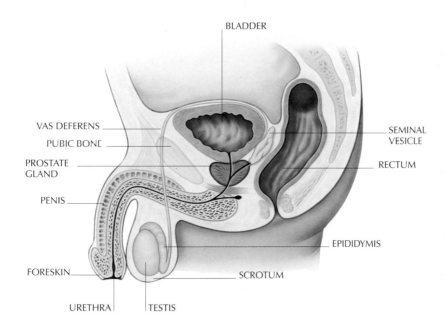

BLADDER

VAS DEFERENS

PUBIC BONE

PROSTATE GLAND

PENIS

SEMINAL VESICLE

RECTUM

EPIDIDYMIS

FORESKIN

SCROTUM

URETHRA

TESTIS

THE MALE REPRODUCTIVE SYSTEM

Testes

The testes serve the same purpose as do ovaries in the female. In fact, they arise from the same embryonic cells. In the male fetus, the testes are developed in the abdomen and descend into the scrotum about two months prior to birth. The testes produce sperm and testosterone (male sex hormone).

Scrotum

The scrotum holds the testes and provides temperature control for them. In order to produce mature sperm, the testes must be about 1.8°F cooler than the body temperature.

Varicocele is the dilation of a vein in the scrotum that causes the pressure to build in the testicles impairing sperm development. This is one of the most common causes of male infertility. This condition is often painless and undetected.

Epididymis

Epididymis is a tightly coiled tube that sits on the top of the testes where sperm is stored to mature before released. If uncoiled, the length of the epididymis would stretch out to about 20 feet long.

Vas Deferens

Vas deferens, also known as the sperm tube, is a long curvy tube that begins at the tail end of the epididymis and winds its way into the abdominal region. The vas deferens acts as a conduit for sperm release. The popular male contraceptive method of vasectomy involves removal of a small section of each vas deferens to stop the sperm from passing through; although more modern techniques involve blocking the tube rather than cutting it.

Seminal Vesicles

Seminal vesicles are paired glands that are located behind the bladder. They produce seminal fluids, which constitute much of the semen.

Prostate Gland

Slightly larger than a size of a walnut, the prostate gland is located at the base of the bladder. The main function of the prostate gland is also to produce fluids to add to the semen.

Urethra

The urethra is a tube that is about 8 inches long, which reaches from the bladder, through the prostate gland and to the end of the penis. The urethra has a dual function: to carry the semen and the urine to the external environment.

Penis

The penis is the external male sexual organ that is composed of sponge-like erectile tissues, blood vessels, the urethra, and sinus cavities. It delivers sperm to the vagina and also eliminates urine.

Impotence is a sexual dysfunction that is the inability to achieve and maintain the erection of the penis.

The Sperm

While women are born with all the eggs they'll use in their lifetime, sperm are constantly generated. Sperm are produced each day, about some 200 million of them, but it takes about 70 days for immature sperm to become fully mature. This is one of the reasons why, in Oriental Medicine, a man should be treated about three months prior to his donation of sperm.

During intercourse, after the semen is ejaculated into the vagina, the sperm has to get through the cervical canal and to the uterine cavity. Once in the uterine cavity, the sperm have to swim forward a distance that is comparatively as far as swimming from one end of Lake Michigan to the other. The sperms' difficult journey does not end there. The most daunting task of all is to find the egg and break through its outer layer to fertilize it. It takes the strongest of all sperm to win this race!

FEMALE REPRODUCTIVE ANATOMY

This section will cover the basic anatomy of the female reproductive system and explain how the system works.

Ovaries

The ovaries are a pair of almond-sized sexual organs located by the uterus. They contain eggs that are released monthly to be fertilized by the sperm in the fallopian tubes. At birth, the ovaries contain all the eggs that a woman will ovulate in her lifetime. The ovaries and the eggs are formed at around the fourth or fifth month of fetal development.

At birth, the ovaries contain about 1 million eggs. By puberty, at the onset of menarche, there are about 300,000 to 400,000 eggs remaining to develop and ovulate in monthly cycles until menopause.

Egg selection and maturation process is called folliculogenesis. It takes about one year for selected follicles to develop into mature follicles, which release the eggs at ovulation. How the follicle selection process takes place and why many of the follicles are left to die is still unknown by modern science.

Eggs contain 23 chromosomes which combine with sperm to make an embryo.

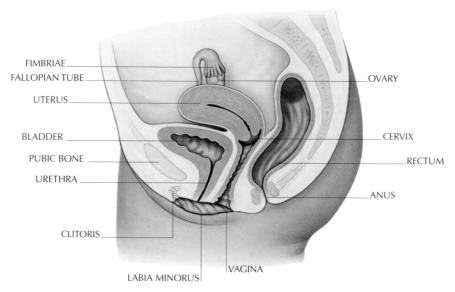

FIMBRIAE
FALLOPIAN TUBE
UTERUS
BLADDER
PUBIC BONE
URETHRA
CLITORIS
LABIA MINORUS
VAGINA
OVARY
CERVIX
RECTUM
ANUS

THE FEMALE REPRODUCTIVE SYSTEM

Fallopian Tubes

Fallopian tubes are two tubes connecting the uterus to the ovaries. The tubes are not connected to the ovaries but the fimbriae (finger-like ends at the end of each fallopian tube) sweep up the egg when it's ovulated from the follicle in the ovary. Most of the time, fertilization of the egg occurs in the fallopian tube. The embryo then is carried out through the fallopian tube to the uterus. In transit, the embryo goes through rapid cell division and becomes a blastocyst, with differentiating cell bodies to become the fetus and the placenta. It takes about five days for the embryo to reach the uterus for implantation.

Uterus

The uterus is where the embryo implants and grows. A pear-shaped organ, it is lined with endometrium, which supports and nourishes the embryo through fetal development until birth. The endometrium develops and sheds every month with the rise and fall of the hormone changes. It is the shedding of the endometrial lining that results in menstruation. When a woman is pregnant, this pear-sized organ can grow to be the size of a watermelon!

The uterus comes in different sizes shapes and orientations. Some women require surgical correction in order for pregnancy to occur. Abnormal growths, such as polyps and fibroids, that can cause infertility, may also be found in the uterus.

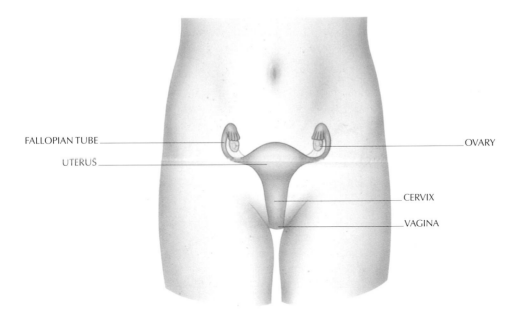

FALLOPIAN TUBE

UTERUS

OVARY

CERVIX

VAGINA

THE FEMALE REPRODUCTIVE SYSTEM

Cervix

The cervix is the lower end of the uterus, where the cervical mucus is produced in response to an increase in estrogen. The secretion of cervical mucus is very important because it helps to transport sperm into the uterine cavity.

Our cervical environment is usually acidic. It is this secretion of cervical mucus that makes the cervical environment less acidic. Sperm live better in this type of environment. This is one of the reasons why the timing of intercourse is so important in achieving pregnancy. The cervix also filters out the abnormal sperm, preventing entrance into the uterus and prevents the baby from falling out of the uterus before it is delivered.

Vagina

This is the passage that connects the cervix to the vulva (the outer genitalia). During intercourse, semen is delivered to the vagina before it enters the cervix. Glands present in the vaginal wall are stimulated to produce fluids during intercourse to make sex more enjoyable. The vagina is highly elastic and can stretch to many times its original size during birth.

APPENDIX D: Acupuncture and Fertility Research

The following table contains some of the research supporting acupuncture and fertility.

STUDY	ABSTRACT	CONCLUSION
Influence of acupuncture on the pregnancy rate in patients who undergo assisted reproduction therapy Wolfgang E. Paulus, M.D., Mingmin Zhang, M.D., Erwin Strehler, M.D.,Imam El-Danasouri, Ph.D., and Karl Sterzik, M.D. Christian-Lauritzen-Institut, Ulm, Germany. *Fertility and Sterility®* 2002; 77: 721-4. ©2002 by American Society for Reproductive Medicine. Published by Elsevier Science Inc.	The aim of this study was to evaluate the effect of acupuncture on the pregnancy rate in assisted reproduction therapy (ART) by comparing a group of 80 patients receiving acupuncture treatment shortly before and after embryo transfer with a control group of 80 patients receiving no acupuncture.	**Results** Clinical pregnancies were documented in 34 of 80 patients (42.5 percent) in the acupuncture group, whereas pregnancy rate was only 26.3 percent (21 out of 80 patients) in the control group. **Conclusion** Acupuncture seems to be a useful tool for improving pregnancy rate after ART. (*Fertility and Sterility®*2002; 77:721-4. ©2002 by American Society for Reproductive Medicine)
Acupuncture normalizes dysfunction of hypothalamic-pituitary-ovarian axis Bo-Ying Chen, M.D. Professor of Neurobiology, Institute of Acupuncture and Department of Neurobiology, Shanghai Medical University *Acupuncture & Electro-Therapeutics Res., Int. J.* 1997; 22: 97-108.	Ten patients with anovulation were treated with electroacupuncture (EA) on day 10 of their cycle. Five more women served as controls. Additional study involved the use of electro-acupuncture on rats.	1. EA induces maturation and exfoliation of vaginal epithelium cell and enhances blood level of E2. 2. EA promotes enlargement of adrenals and enhances activity of adrenal AgNORs as well as blood level of corticosterone. 3. EA decreases the level of hypothalamic GnRH, pituitary LH and increases the contents of hypothalamic and pituitary ß-endorphin.
Reduction of blood flow impedance in the uterine arteries of infertile women with electro-acupuncture Elisabet Stener-Victorin, Urban Waldenström, Sven A. Andersson and Matts Wikland, Sweden. *Source:* European Society for Human Reproduction and Embryology	The pulsatility index of women before and after a course of electro-acupuncture treatments was measured.	Pulsatility index dropped significantly after the treatments, and 10–14 days after the last treatment.
Acupuncture treatment for infertile women undergoing intracytoplasmic sperm injection Sandra L. Emmons, M.D. and Phillip Patton, M.D. *Medical Acupuncture: A Journal for Physicians by Physicians.* Spring/Summer 2000; 12(2).	**Design, setting, and patients** Prospective case series of six women receiving intracytoplasmic sperm injection and acupuncture along with agents for ovarian stimulation. **Main outcome measures** Number of follicles retrieved, conception, and pregnancy past the first trimester before and after acupuncture treatment.	**Results** No pregnancies occurred in the non-acupuncture cycles. Three women produced more follicles with acupuncture treatment (mean, 11.3 vs 3.9 prior to acupuncture; p = 0.005). All three women conceived, but only one pregnancy lasted past the first trimester. **Conclusion** Acupuncture may be a useful adjunct to gonadotropin therapy to produce follicles in women undergoing in-vitro fertilization.

STUDY	ABSTRACT	CONCLUSION
Does acupuncture treatment affect sperm density in males with very low sperm count? A pilot study Siterman S, Eltes F, Wolfson V, Lederman H, Bartoov B. Institute of Chinese Medicine, Tel Aviv, Israel. *Andrologia.* 2000 Jan; 32(1): 31–9.	Semen samples of 20 patients with a history of azoospermia were examined by light microscope and scanning electron microscope, with which a microsearch for spermatozoa was carried out. Examinations were performed before and one month after acupuncture treatment. The control group comprised 20 untreated males who underwent two semen examinations within a period of 2–4 months and had initial andrological profiles similar to those of the experimental group.	No changes in any of the parameters examined were observed in the control group. A definite increase in sperm count was detected in the ejaculates of 10 (67 percent) of the 15 azoospermic patients. It is concluded that acupuncture may be a useful, nontraumatic treatment for males with very poor sperm density.
Effect of acupuncture on sperm parameters of males suffering from subfertility related to low sperm quality Siterman S, Eltes F, Wolfson V, Zablu-dovsky N, Bartoov B. Institute of Chinese Medicine, Tel Aviv, Israel. *Arch Androl.* 1997 Sep–Oct; 39(2): 155–61.	Semen samples of 16 acupuncture-treated subfertile patients were analyzed before and 1 month after treatment (twice a week for 5 weeks). In parallel, semen samples of 16 control untreated subfertile males were examined. Two specimens were taken from the control group at an interval of 2–8 months.	The fertility index increased significantly (p < or = 0.05) following improvement in total functional sperm fraction, percentage of viability, total motile spermatozoa per ejaculate, and integrity of the axonema (p < or = 0.05), which occurred upon treatment.
Quantitative evaluation of spermatozoa ultrastructure after acupuncture treatment for idiopathic male infertility Jian Pei, Ph.D., Erwin Strehler, M.D., Ulrich Noss, M.D., Markus Abt, Ph.D., Paola Piomboni, Ph.D., Baccio Baccetti, Ph.D., Karl Sterzik, M.D. Christian-Lauritzen-Institut, Ulm, IVF center Munich, Germany, and Department of General Biology, University of Siena, Siena, Italy. *Fertility and Sterility®* 2005 July; 84(1): 141-7.	The objective was to evaluate the ultramorphologic sperm features of idiopathic infertile men after acupuncture therapy. Forty men with idiopathic oligospermia, asthenospermia, or teratozoospermia were enrolled in a prospective controlled study. Twenty eight of the patients received acupuncture twice a week over a period of five weeks The samples from the treatment group were randomized with semen samples from the 12 men in the untreated control group. Quantitative analysis by transmission electron microscopy (TEM) was used to evaluate the samples, using the mathematical formula based on submicro-scopic characteristics.	**Results** Statistical evaluation of the TEM data showed a statistically significant increase after acupuncture in the percentage and number of sperm without ultrastructural defects in the total ejaculates. A statistically significant improvement was detected in acrosome position and shape, nuclear shape, axonemal pattern and shape, and accessory fibers of sperm organelles. However, specific sperm pathologies in the form of apoptosis, immaturity, and necrosis showed no statistically significant changes between the control and treatment groups before and after treatment. **Conclusion** The treatment of idiopathic male infertility could benefit from employing acupuncture. A general improvement of sperm quality, specifically in the ultrastructural integrity of spermatozoa, was seen after acupuncture, although we did not identify specific sperm pathologies that could be particularly sensitive to this therapy.

Bibliography

American Institute of Stress. *America's Number 1 Health Problem.* http://www.stress.org/americas.htm Accessed February 2008.

American Society of Reproductive Medicine. *Patient Fact Sheet: Weight and Fertility.* http://www.asrm.org/Patients/FactSheets/weightfertility.pdf Accessed February 2007.

Beinfield, H. and Korngold, E. *Between Heaven and Earth: A Guide to Chinese Medicine.* New York NY: BALLANTINE BOOKS, 1991.

Bensky, D., Clavey, S., Stoger, E., with Gamble, A. *Chinese Herbal Medicine: Materia Medica, Third Edition.* Seattle WA: EASTLAND PRESS, 2004.

Berga, S. Recovery of ovarian activity in women with functional hypothalamic amenorrhea who were treated with cognitive behavior therapy. *Fertility and Sterility* (2003) 80(4), 976–981.

Carr, B.R. and Blackwell, R.E. *Textbook of Reproductive Medicine: Second Edition.* Stamford CT: APPLETON AND LANGE, 1998.

Cassidy, A. *et al.* Biological effects of a diet of soy protein rich in isoflavones on the menstrual cycle of premenopausal women. *Am J Clin Nutr* (1994) 60, 333–340.

Chang, J. *The Tao of Love and Sex: The Ancient Chinese Way to Ecstasy.* NewYork NY: PENGUIN BOOKS, 1977.

Chavarro, J.E. *et al.* A prospective study of dairy foods intake and anovulatory infertility. *Human Reprod* (2007) 22, 1340–1347.

Chen, T.H., Chang S.P., Tsai C.F., Juang K.D. Prevalence of depressive and anxiety disorders in an assisted reproductive technique clinic. *Human Reprod* (2004) 19(10), 2313–2318.

Chopra, D. *The Seven Spiritual Laws of Success.* San Rafael CA, AMBER-ALLEN PUBLISHING, 2007.

Cohen, K.S. *The Way of Qigong: The Art and Science of Chinese Energy Healing.* New York NY: BALLANTINE BOOKS, 1997.

Deadman, P., AlKhafaji, M., with Baker, K. *A Manual of Acupuncture.* Vista CA: EASTLAND PRESS, 1999.

Desikachar, T.K.V. *The Heart of Yoga: Developing a Personal Practice.* Rochester NY: INNER TRADITIONS, 1999.

Farrow, J.T. *et al.* Breath suspension during the transcendental meditation technique. *Psychosom Med* (1982) 44, 133–153.

Feinberg, R. *Healing Syndrome "O": A Strategic Guide to Fertility, Polycystic Ovaries, and Insulin Imbalance.* New York NY: PENGUIN GROUP, 2004.

Frawley, D. *Yoga & Ayurveda: Self-Healing and Self-Realization.* Twin Lakes, WI: LOTUS PRESS, 1999.

Ganmaa, D. *et al.* The possible role of female sex hormones in milk from pregnant cows in the development of breast, ovarian and corpus uteri cancers. *Med Hypotheses* (2005) 65, 1028–37.

Gesink Law, D. Obesity and time to pregnancy. *Human Reprod* (2007) 22, 414–20.

Hale, G. *The Practical Encyclopedia of Feng Shui.* London: HERMES HOUSE, 2003.

Hellstrom, W.J.G. ed. *Male Infertility and Sexual Dysfunction.* New York NY: SPRINGER, 1997.

Jevning, R. *et al.* The physiology of meditation: a review. A wakeful hypometabolic integrated response. *Neurosci Biobehav Sci* (1992) 16, 415–24.

Kabat-Zinn, J. The clinical use of mindfulness meditation for the self-regulation of chronic pain. *J Behav Med* (1985) 8, 163–90.

Kaptchuck, T.J. *The Web that Has No Weaver: Understanding Chinese Medicine.* Lincolnwood IL: MCGRAW HILL/CONTEMPORARY BOOKS, 2000.

Klonoff-Cohen, H. A prospective study of stress among women undergoing in vitro fertilization or gamete intrafallopian transfer. *Fertility and Sterility* (2001) 76, 675–87.

Kriyananda, G. *The Spiritual Science of Kriya Yoga.* Chicago IL: THE TEMPLE OF KRIYA YOGA, 1992.

Kushner, H. *When Bad Things Happen to Good People.* London, HARPER PERENNIAL, 1983.

Lemaire, G. Activation of alpha- and beta-estrogen receptors by persistent pesticides in reporter cell lines. *Life Sci* (2006) 79, 1160–69.

Lu, L.J. *et al.* Effects of an isoflavone-free soy diet on ovarian hormones in premenopausal women. *J. Clin Endocrinol Metab* (2001) 86, 3045–52.

Lu, L.J. Effects of soya consumption for one month on steroid hormones in premenopausal women: implications for breast cancer risk reduction. *Cancer Epidemiol Biomarkers* (1996) 1, 63–70.

Lyttleton, J. *Treatment of Infertility with Chinese Medicine.* Edinburgh: CHURCHILL LIVINGSTONE, 2004.

Maciocia, G. *The Foundations of Chinese Medicine.* Edinburgh: CHURCHILL LIVINGSTONE, 1989.

Maciocia, G. *Obstertrics and Gynecology in Chinese Medicine.* Edinburgh: CHURCHILL LIVINGSTONE, 1998.

Malekinejad, H. *et al.* Naturally occurring estrogens in processed milk and in raw milk (from gestated cows). *J Agric Food Chem* (2006) 54, 9785–91.

Morris, S.N. *et al.* Effects of lifetime exercise on the outcome of in vitro fertilization. *Obstet Gynecol* (2006) 108, 938–45.

Nettleton, J.A. Straight Talk about Eating Fish During Pregnancy. *www.alaskaseafood.org* (2002) Accessed May 2007.

O'Halloran, J.P. *et al.* Hormonal control in a state of decreased activation: potentiation of arginine vasopressin secretion. *Physiology and Behavior* (1985) 35, 591–595.

Pal, G.K. *et al.* Effect of short-term practice of breathing exercises on autonomic functions in normal human volunteers. *Indian J Med Res* (2004) 120, 115–21.

Pansky, B. *Review of Medical Embryology.* New York NY: MACMILLAN, 1982.

Pitchford, P. *Healing with Whole Foods: Asian Traditions and Modern Nutrition,Third Edition.* Berkeley CA: NORTH ATLANTIC BOOKS, 2002.

Reid, D.P. *The Tao of Health, Sex and Longevity: A Modern Practical Guide to the Ancient Way.* New York NY: FIRESIDE, 1989.

Sallman, M. *et al.* Reduced fertility among overweight and obese men. *Epidemiology.* 5 (2006) pp. 520–3.

Sternberg, E. *Changing the Face of Medicine,* Accessed March 2008. *http://www.nlm.nih.gov/changingthefaceofmedicine/exhibition/*

Tierra, M. *Planetary Herbology.* Twin Lakes WI: LOTUS PRESS, 1992.

Tiwari, M. *A Life of Balance.* Rochester NY: HEALING ARTS PRESS, 1995.

Too, L. *Essential Feng Shui: A Step-by-Step Guide to Enhancing Your Relationships, Health and Prosperity.* New York NY: BALLANTINE WELLSPRING, 1998.

Wang, K *et al.* Psychological characteristics and marital quality of infertile women registered for in vitro fertilization-intracytoplasmic sperm injection in China. *Fertility and Sterility* (2007) 87, Issue 4, Pages 792–798.

Weschler, T. *Taking Charge of Your Fertility: The Definitive Guide to Natural Birth Control, Pregnancy Achievement, and Reproductive Health,* Revised Edition. New York NY: QUILL, 2002.

Wile, D. *Art of the Bedchamber: The Chinese Sexual Yoga Classic including Women's Solo Meditation Texts.* Albany NY: SUNY, 1992.

Wiseman, N. and Ellis, A. *Fundamentals of Chinese Medicine, Revised Edition.* Brookline MA: PARADIGM PUBLICATIONS, 1996.

Zettnersan, Master C. *Taoist Bedroom Secrets.* Twin Lakes WI: LOTUS PRESS, 2002.

Index